VIROLOGY MONOGRAPHS

DIE VIRUSFORSCHUNG IN EINZELDARSTELLUNGEN

CONTINUING/FORTFÜHRUNG VON
HANDBOOK OF VIRUS RESEARCH
HANDBUCH DER VIRUSFORSCHUNG
FOUNDED BY/BEGRÜNDET VON
R. DOERR

EDITED BY/HERAUSGEGEBEN VON

S. GARD · C. HALLAUER · K. F. MEYER

9

1971

SPRINGER-VERLAG

NEW YORK   WIEN

AFRICAN SWINE FEVER VIRUS

BY

W. R. HESS

BLUETONGUE VIRUS

BY

P. G. HOWELL AND D. W. VERWOERD

1971

SPRINGER-VERLAG

NEW YORK   WIEN

ISBN 0-387-81006-4
ISBN 3-211-81006-4

African Swine Fever Virus

By

W. R. Hess

Plum Island Animal Disease Laboratory, Animal Disease and Parasite
Research Division,
Agricultural Research Service, United States Department of Agriculture,
P.O. Box 848, Greenport, New York 11944, U.S.A.

With 1 Figure

Table of Contents

I. Introduction 2

II. History 2

III. Classification and Nomenclature 4

IV. Properties of the Virus 7
    A. Morphology 7
    B. Chemical Composition 7
    C. Antigenic Composition 9
    D. Effects of Physical and Chemical Agents on Infectivity 11

V. Cultivation in Cell Cultures 13
    A. Host-cell Range 13
    B. Virus Reproductive Cycle in Cell Cultures 14
    C. Replication and Cytopathogenesis in Cell Cultures 15
        1. Light Microscopy 15
        2. Electron Microscopy 15

VI. Interaction with Organisms 17
    A. Host Range 17
    B. Pathogenesis in Domestic Swine 19
    C. Clinical Manifestations and Pathology in Domestic Swine 21
    D. Immunity 23
    E. Virus Modification in Domestic Swine 24
    F. Diagnosis 25
    G. Epizootiology 26

References 27

Addendum 33

I. Introduction

The causative agent of African swine fever (ASF) is an icosahedral virus 175 to 215 mμ in diameter. It is sensitive to lipid solvents and contains deoxyribonucleic acid (DNA). Thus far, it appears to have no close relatives among other viruses that infect mammals. It has apparently existed for a very long time in wild swine indigenous to Africa, for with them it has established an ideal host-parasite relationship in which prolonged infection occurs without signs of disease. In fact, the existence of the virus came to light only after domestic swine of European origin were brought into areas inhabited by wart hogs. Although the precise mode of transmission from wild swine is obscure, the virus spreads readily among domestic swine and produces a peracute disease with mortality approaching 100 per cent. Since the swine industry is quite sparse in such areas, the outbreaks are largely self-limiting. Each outbreak usually represents a new incursion of the virus from its natural reservoir. This continues to be the pattern of most outbreaks in Africa, and until recently the peracute infection which prevails under these conditions has been regarded as the usual form of the disease in domestic swine. However, ASF has spread to Europe and in some areas has become enzootic in domestic swine. In these areas, acute, subacute, and chronic infections are common and the mortality is somewhat reduced. Its resemblance to classical swine fever (American hog cholera and European swine fever) has become more pronounced, and differential diagnosis in the field is seldom possible. In addition, inapparent carriers and arthropod vectors have become increasingly important in the maintenance and spread of the disease. That which has been regarded as an emerging disease capable of completely destroying domestic swine populations must now also be regarded as an evolving disease tending toward a more satisfactory accommodation to a newly acquired host. There is little comfort in this knowledge, for as the disease has become milder, it has also become more insidious and prospects of effective control have accordingly diminished. Furthermore, as long as the natural reservoirs exist, there is always the threat of new incursions of fully virulent strains of the virus. From what is known of the immunology of ASF, a new strain of virus could be as devastating to domestic swine in an enzootic area as the established strain was when it first appeared. A safe and effective vaccine is not yet available, and it appears likely that a number of questions concerning the obscure immunology of ASF must be answered before development of a suitable prophylactic agent will be possible. Some of the answers will perhaps be found by studying the pathogenesis of the disease in its various forms, and others must ultimately be revealed in the structure, composition, and mode of replication of the virus particle. Studies along these lines made possible through the application of cell culture methods have appeared only since 1960. A substantial portion of this review is devoted to the analysis of these recent studies and includes information available as of May 1969.

II. History

Although the history of ASF up to 1965 has been presented in detail elsewhere (DeTray, 1963; Neitz, 1963; Scott, 1965a), some of the highlights are reiterated here to give proper perspective to information that has since appeared.

With good reason, ASF has frequently been referred to as Montgomery's disease. He described the disease, established its viral nature, determined it to be immunologically distinct from classical swine fever, studied the survival of the virus under a variety of environmental conditions, explored methods of transmission and immunization, studied the host range, and indicated the possible role of wild swine in maintaining the disease in nature (MONTGOMERY, 1921). These observations were made in Kenya during the period from 1910 to 1915 in outbreaks involving 1,366 swine with a mortality of 98.9 per cent.

During the ensuing forty-two years outbreaks of ASF were reported in various areas south of the Sahara in Africa. The studies during this period confirmed and enlarged upon Montgomery's findings, scored the immunological peculiarities of the disease, and emphasized its potential threat to the world's swine industry. The wart hog *(Phacochoerus)* and bush pig *(Potamochoerus)* were found to harbor the virus in nature (STEYN, 1932; DE KOCK et al., 1940; HAMMOND and DETRAY, 1955), but the mechanism of transmission to domestic swine remained obscure. On at least two occasions during this period, virus was imported for study in Europe, and the immunologic distinction between ASF and classical swine fever was convincingly demonstrated (MONTGOMERY, 1921; GEIGER, 1937). Domestic swine that had survived infection and were refractory to challenge with the homologous virus isolate were occasionally encountered and studied (WALKER, 1933; STEYN, 1932; DE KOCK et al., 1940; DETRAY, 1957a), but the numbers were never sufficient to enable extensive investigation of the condition, nor were antibodies demonstrable by the serologic test procedures used. Because animals refractory to one virus isolate seldom withstood challenge with heterologous isolates, it was concluded that more than one, and perhaps many, immunologic types existed. All efforts to produce immunity with virus rendered noninfectious by physical or chemical means were unsuccessful. The refractory state was invariably preceded by infection, and in most instances, the so-called immune animals were in fact virus carriers (DETRAY, 1957a). Subacute and chronic infections were rarely encountered, and in practically all reports from Africa, ASF was described as a peracute, fulminating disease with mortality closely approaching 100 per cent. The alarming potential of the disease was clearly apparent.

Despite the ominous warnings, concern about ASF in most major swine-producing countries was aroused only after the disease appeared in Portugal in 1957. This first incursion of the disease outside the continent of Africa was apparently eradicated (MANSO RIBEIRO et al., 1958), but it recurred in Portugal in 1960 and spread to Spain (ANONYMOUS, 1961). Fortunately, during this period, a major breakthrough in research on ASF was achieved in Kenya. The virus was successfully propagated in swine bone marrow and buffy coat cell cultures (MALMQUIST and HAY, 1960). In such cultures, erythrocytes present became adsorbed on the surfaces of infected macrophages. This reaction became the basis of an *in vitro* test which served as a convenient means of detecting the virus and distinguishing between ASF and classical swine fever. The test has been of tremendous value in identifying the disease in Portugal and Spain (C. SANCHEZ BOTIJA and R. SANCHEZ BOTIJA, 1965) and more recently in France and Italy.

In early 1964, outbreaks of ASF were reported in France along the Pyrennes Mountains and in the Department of Brittany (LARENAUDIE et al., 1964). The disease was apparently eradicated by a drastic slaughter program in which all infected and exposed swine were eliminated without distinction being made between ASF and classical swine fever. In April of 1967 the disease was reported in Italy occurring in swine in the vicinity of Rome. Again a drastic slaugther program was credited with eliminating the disease. However, at the time of this writing, ASF is still present in Portugal and Spain and has again been reported in Italy.

III. Classification and Nomenclature

It is believed that there is more than one immunologic type of ASF virus (WALKER, 1933; GEIGER, 1937; HENNING, 1956; MALMQUIST, 1963; STONE and HESS, 1965; COGGINS, 1968a). Because there is as yet no well-established or generally accepted method for distinguishing the various serotypes, virus stocks will be referred to here either as isolates, or if they are known to originate from particular isolates, but differ from them in some property (e.g. virulence) or by virtue of adaptation to another host (e.g. cell cultures), they will be designated as strains of the parent isolates.

There are more than fifty isolates on hand in various laboratories. Many were obtained from domestic swine in Africa and were from outbreaks so separated in time and/or locality as to rule out or at least obscure any continuity among them. Others were isolated from wild swine collected at random or in some instances collected in the vicinity of an outbreak in domestic swine. Finally, several virus isolates were collected in Portugal, Spain, France, and Italy. With the possible exception of the 1957 isolate from Portugal, all of the European isolates are probably derived from the same parent stock.

Although they may differ somewhat in virulence, all of the isolates produce clinically recognizable swine fever in domestic swine and cause hemadsorption (HAd) in swine buffy coat cultures. There is strong cross-reactivity among all ASF virus isolates that have thus far been tested by complement-fixation (CF), agar gel diffusion precipitation (AGDP), or fluorescent-antibody (FA) techniques (HESS et al., 1965; STONE and HESS, 1965; COGGINS and HEUSCHELE, 1966; HEUSCHELE et al., 1966; BOULANGER et al., 1967a, b, c). All that have been tested with antisera of classical swine fever by any of these techniques (MALMQUIST, 1963; COWAN, 1961; HEUSCHELE et al., 1966; BOULANGER et al., 1967c), or have been subjected to cross-immunity tests in swine (DeTRAY and SCOTT, 1955; DeLAY and CARBREY, 1963; HAAG et al., 1965) have proven to be immunologically distinct from classical swine fever.

At least five isolates or their cell culture-adapted strains have been examined by electron microscopy, used in nucleic acid determinations, and subjected to the effects of heat, pH, and lipid solvents. Among them were isolates from both Europe and Africa, and the findings with all were virtually the same. The present contemplation of the classification of ASF virus is based largely on these findings.

On the basis of sensitivity to lipid solvents, the HAd property, size, morphology, and mode of replication, it was thought that ASF virus might be related to the large myxoviruses (ANDREWES, 1962; HESS et al., cited by DeTRAY, 1963; BREESE and DE BOER, 1966). This possibility was excluded when the virus was found to contain DNA (HAAG et al., 1965; PLOWRIGHT et al., 1966; ADLDINGER et al., 1966; BREESE and DE BOER, 1967).

Of the DNA-containing mammalian viruses having the status of a major group or family in present virus classification schemes, only the herpesvirus bear a substantial resemblance to ASF virus. Both are sensitive to lipid solvents, and it has been pointed out (BREESE and DE BOER, 1966) that herpes simplex virus (CHITWOOD and BRACKEN, 1964), infectious laryngotracheitis virus (WATRACH, 1962) and human cytomegalovirus (PINKERTON et al., 1964) have morphological appearances similar to ASF virus when seen in thin sections. However, at no time in its growth cycle is ASF virus seen in the nucleus of the infected host cell. Its entire assembly appears to take place in the cytoplasm. Furthermore, ASF virus has not been shown to have the distinctive capsid structure of the herpesvirus group, nor is its stability at low pH (PLOWRIGHT and PARKER, 1967) compatible with the properties of that group of viruses.

The Lucké frog kidney tumor virus and other closely related polyhedral cytoplasmic viruses of amphibia have such a striking resemblance to ASF virus when seen in thin sections (BREESE and DE BOER, 1967; LUNGER and CAME, 1966) that a search for possible relationships among them seemed warranted. In each instance, the viruses contain DNA, multiply in the cytoplasm, emerge from the cell in a similar manner and are sensitive to lipid solvents. However, it was found that ASF virus and the cytoplasmic frog viruses are not serologically related nor do they share a common host range (CAME and DARDIRI, 1969). It is noteworthy that neither ASF virus nor the frog viruses (FV 1 and FV 3) appear to be capable of stimulating the production of neutralizing antibodies (CAME, personal communication; DE BOER, 1967 a, b; DE BOER et al., 1969).

Morphological similarities between ASF virus and Tipula iridescent virus have been noted and an effort has been made to delineate and compare the capsid structure of the two viruses (ALMEIDA et al., 1967). It is suggested that both are of the compound cubic type and have icosahedral forms built up of regular subunits in a triangular arrangement and stabilized by the addition of outer membranes. Lymphocystis virus of fish (WEISSENBERG, 1965) is also of very similar morphology (ZWILLENBERG and WOLF, 1968), but unlike ASF virus and the frog viruses, neither Tipula iridescent virus nor lymphocystis virus have been observed to acquire an additional membrane during passage through the cytoplasmic membrane of the host cell (BIRD, 1962; ZWILLENBERG and ZWILLENBERG, 1963).

At present, ASF virus appears to be unique among the mammalian viruses. It does have many characteristics in common with the polyhedral cytoplasmic viruses from amphibia, and though there is a lack of serological relationship and a marked difference in host range, nothing has been revealed thus far that would preclude taxonomic association of these viruses at the level of a family. Nevertheless, until their capsid structures have been resolved and found to be similar, such association is premature.

During the preparation of this review, a report appeared (LUCAS and CARNERO, 1968) in which it was concluded that the aggregate of characteristics of ASF virus excludes it from all of the virus families thus far included in the classification scheme recommended by the Provisional Committee for Nomenclature of Viruses (Proposals and Recommendations of the PROVISIONAL COMMITTEE FOR NOMENCLATURE OF VIRUSES, 1965). It was proposed that a new family of which ASF virus is the only known representative be established and designated as

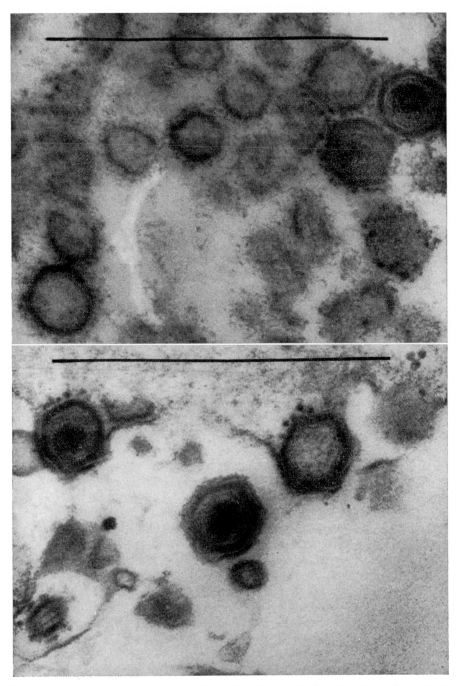

Fig. 1. African swine fever virus in swine kidney cells 48 hours after infection. Upper: Formation in cytoplasm. Mature virus has dense central core and multilayered outer shell. Lower: Virus emerging from cell by budding. An outer membrane is acquired. Magnification mark = 1 μ
(Courtesy Sydney S. Breese, Jr., Plum Island Animal Disease Laboratory)

Asupesviridae (from *Africanae suis pestis viridae*). This proposal may prove to be entirely justified. If, however, the family is to be defined according to the criteria recommended for this system of classification, it may be well to withhold a decision until the capsid structure of ASF virus has been clearly resolved.

IV. Properties of the Virus
A. Morphology

African swine fever virus, as visualized by electron microscopy in thin sections of infected cells (BREESE and DE BOER, 1966; HAAG *et al.*, 1966) appears in the cytoplasm as particles, 175—215 mµ in diameter. The virion consists of a dense central nucleoid 72—89 mµ in diameter surrounded by an electron-lucent area 35 mµ in width and enclosed in a distinct hexagonal outer shell (Fig. 1). As the particle emerges from the cell by budding, it acquires an outer envelope composed of material from the cytoplasmic membrane. Particles sectioned through the apparent center of the structure display a maximum of nucleoid and are hexagonal in shape. Particles sectioned through regions with less nucleoid are often pentagonal. From this it is inferred that the virion is probably icosahedral in form.

In cell spread preparations examined by the negative-staining technique, a second type of particle has been revealed (ALMEIDA *et al.*, 1967). It lacks a distinct bounding membrane and is built up of regular repeating subunits in triangular arrangement. It is suggested that such particles are the collapsed remains of icosahedral shells and are indicative of the capsid structure of the virus particle as it appears when free of its stabilizing outer membranes. The interpretation is strengthened somewhat by the fact that Tipula iridescent virus which closely resembles ASF virus when seen in thin sections also yields particles of a similar nature in cell spread preparations. Also, a suggestion of this capsid structure was occasionally seen in particles of the stable hexagonal types. On the basis of these observations, it is suggested that ASF virus is of the compound cubic type having icosahedral symmetry. It is further stated that the number of capsomers comprising the capsid of the virus is likely to be of the order of 812. Although the inferences drawn in this study may be entirely correct, it is hoped that they may be substantiated by a more convincing resolution of the fine structure of the identifiable stable virion.

B. Chemical Composition

Inclusion bodies formed within the cytoplasm of cells infected with ASF virus stained specifically for DNA by the Feulgen and acridine orange techniques (HAAG and LARENAUDIE, 1965). This first indication of the type of nucleic acid in ASF virus was soon amply confirmed. Viral synthesis was inhibited by 5-iodo-2'-deoxyuridine (IUDR), 5-bromo-2'-deoxyuridine (BUDR), and 5-fluoro-2'-deoxyuridine (FUDR), and in each instance inhibition was reversed by addition of thymidine (HAAG *et al.*, 1965; PLOWRIGHT *et al.*, 1966; MOULTON and COGGINS, 1968a). Hydroxyurea (HU) also had an inhibitory effect (MOULTON and COGGINS, 1968a). Its effect on the synthesis of ASF virus is of particular interest (BREESE and DE BOER, 1969) and will be discussed later in connection with the growth cycle of the virus. Incorporation of thymidine-^{3}H in developing inclusions has been demonstrated (PLOWRIGHT *et al.*, 1966; VIGÁRIO *et al.*, 1967; MOULTON and

COGGINS, 1968a). Definitive proof was supplied by extraction of an infectious nucleic acid (ADLDINGER et al., 1966) which was resistant to ribonuclease (RNase) but was inactivated by deoxyribonuclease (DNase). The infectious extract had an ultraviolet absorption spectrum and an absorbance-temperature profile characteristic of a double-stranded DNA. Finally, thin sections cut from infected cells embedded in glycol methacrylate were treated with enzymes, stained with uranyl acetate and examined by electron microscopy (BREESE and DE BOER, 1967). The DNA was found to be confined to the central core of the virus particle. Ribonucleic acid was not detected. The same study revealed that the sharply delineated hexagonal outer membrane of the virus contained protein that was digested by pepsin but not by trypsin.

Its sensitivity to lipid solvents (DETRAY, 1963) indicates the presence of lipids that are essential to its structure, and from its mode of egression from the host cell (BREESE and DE BOER, 1966), it may be inferred that some, if not all, of the lipid is in the outermost membrane of the virion. This inference is substantiated by the fact that out of a large group of enzymes among which were pepsin, trypsin, chymotrypsin, papain, nucleases, and lipases only pancreatic lipase brought about a reduction in virus infectivity. The effect of this enzyme was marked (HESS and STONE, unpublished). It appears that the proteinases and DNase are only able to act on ASF virus after its lipid-containing coat has been disrupted.

The application of a number of analytical procedures has been precluded by the inability to obtain pure virus preparations. Purification by extraction with fluorocarbons has been reported (LARENAUDIE et al., 1965). Four cycles of extraction with Freon 113 resulted in a loss of approximately 2 $\log_{10}$ units of infectivity. No estimate of the degree of purification was presented. Similar methods had been tried (HESS, unpublished) but were abandoned because the yields were low, and efforts to concentrate the product by ultracentrifugation or negative-pressure dialysis only led to further losses. The virus remaining after as few as two or three extractions with fluorocarbons was too fragile to withstand the mildest of concentration methods. Perhaps the stability of ASF virus is largely dependent upon the presence of protective substances in its environment. However, it is suspected that the extreme fragility of virus surviving this method of purification is due in part to injury caused by the direct action of the fluorocarbon on the virus particle.

The virus in fluids from infected cell cultures was precipitated by dialysis against low ionic strength (0.01) phosphate buffer at pH 7.5 (STONE and HESS, 1965). Virus recovery was usually better than 99 per cent with purification factors ranging from 100 to 200 as indicated by protein nitrogen analysis. The method served to separate the infectious particles from a number of associated noninfectious antigens, but the virus-containing fraction was not of sufficient purity to enable a precise chemical analysis of the virus. Because a substantial removal of protein is achieved with no appreciable loss of infectious virus, the method may serve well as a first step in the purification.

Efforts to establish some of the fundamental molecular parameters of the virus by ultracentrifugation methods have thus far proved disappointing. An intimate association of the virus with cellular material, a tendency to form aggregates, and an extremely low density may be among the factors responsible for the poor results obtained. Much more work needs to be done in this area.

C. Antigenic Composition

As pointed out previously, there appears to be more than one immunologic type of ASF virus, for it has often been demonstrated that pigs refractory to one virus isolate may not withstand challenge inoculation with an heterologous isolate (WALKER, 1933; GEIGER, 1937; HENNING, 1956; MALMQUIST, 1963). However, cross-immunity tests have lacked systematic design and have been limited in scope. Also, the refractory state exists in the absence of demonstrable neutralizing antibodies, and there is considerable doubt that it is immunity in the classical sense (DeTRAY, 1957a; MALMQUIST, 1963; DE BOER, 1967b). It is now possible with several different isolates to regularly obtain swine that are refractory to challenge inoculation with homologous virus (MALMQUIST, 1962; MANSO RIBEIRO, 1962; SANCHEZ BOTIJA, 1963b; HESS et al., 1965). It is, therefore, feasible for a laboratory that can afford the space, animals, and manpower to conduct reciprocal cross-immunity studies that might unequivocally settle the question of the existence of multiple serotypes among the isolates of ASF virus. Before such a massive effort is undertaken, it might be well to examine and exploit more thoroughly the in vitro methods that have indicated some serologic differences among the isolates.

Cultures of buffy coat and bone marrow cells of swine were readily infected with ASF virus and erythrocytes present in the cultures became adsorbed on the surfaces of infected leukocytes (MALMQUIST and HAY, 1960). This reaction was followed by lysis of the infected leukocytes. It was further shown that serums from pigs that had survived or were chronically infected with ASF virus were often capable of inhibiting the HAd reaction but did not neutralize the cytopathic effect (CPE) produced by infection of the leukocytes. The hemadsorption inhibition (HAdI) reaction appeared to be isolate-specific. Although the HAdI reaction was confirmed, attempts to apply it to more extensive serotyping studies were inconclusive and it was concluded that production of more suitable antisera and standardization of the test procedures were required (STONE and HESS, 1965; COGGINS and HEUSCHELE, 1966). Recently, two modifications of the HAdI test have been developed which apparently overcome the difficulties previously experienced. The procedures are similar in that the buffy coat cultures are prepared by the same method (HESS and DeTRAY, 1960), and the inhibition of HAd is determined only after the majority of leukocytes have become infected and before CPE has occurred. In the first method (CARNERO et al., 1967), the erythrocytes are removed by washing with Hanks' solution two or three days after the cultures are made and before they are infected. The cultures are then infected and the progress of infection is determined by the development of HAd in control cultures to which erythrocytes have been added. In the other method (COGGINS, 1968a) the cultures containing erythrocytes are infected two or three days after preparation, and when the vast majority of leukocytes display HAd, the erythrocytes are removed by a brief washing with distilled water. In both methods, dilutions of the antiserum to be tested are added to the infected erythrocyte-free cultures and held at 37°C for one hour. A suspension of erythrocytes is then added, and the cultures are examined for HAd an hour later.

By means of one of these methods (COGGINS, 1968a) the Hinde, Uganda, and Tengani isolates from Africa and their respective antiserums have been tested reciprocally and found to differ serologically. More recently, it has been determined by the same method that the 1957 and 1960 isolates from Portugal are different (COGGINS, personal communication). It has also been found that an Italian isolate differs from three African isolates but appears to be similar to the Lisbon 1960 and Salamanca isolates (HESS, unpublished).

Although there are no reports of the application of the first method to serologic typing, there is no reason to believe that it would not be at least as satisfactory as the other procedure. It may, in fact, be a more sensitive test because the infected leukocytes are not exposed to the possibly damaging effect of washing with distilled water.

It should be kept in mind that the HAdI reaction probably measures only one of several possible antigenic parameters and may not of itself indicate a difference of sufficient magnitude to be regarded as a true type difference.

It has not been possible to demonstrate hemagglutinin in fluids of infected cell cultures or in tissue extracts from infected animals (MALMQUIST and HAY, 1960). The HAd phenomenon has been examined by electron microscopy (BREESE and HESS, 1966; LARENAUDIE et al., 1967) but a conclusive explanation of the mechanism of the reaction was not revealed. Virus particles were occasionally found in spaces between the infected cell and the adsorbed erythrocytes, but there was little evidence that they served as bridges. Adsorption apparently occurs only on the intact plasma membranes of infected cells, and elution of the erythrocytes takes place when the membrane is disrupted. On the basis of these observations, it was suggested (LARENAUDIE et al., 1967) that an antigen responsible for HAd was formed within the infected cell and acted on the plasma membrane to form binding sites for the red blood cells. Formation of this antigen accompanies viral synthesis but it appears to be independent of the maturation of the virus particle. This is very similar to the mechanism of HAd described for mumps virus (DUC-NGUYEN, 1968). With such a mechanism, it is not difficult to conceive of virus production taking place without formation of hemadsorbing antigen. The segregation and propagation of nonhemadsorbing ASF virus (COGGINS, 1968b) appears to bear this out. Furthermore, an antiserum which is apparently capable of neutralizing homologous virus also inhibits CPE produced by the nonhemadsorbing strain of that virus.

Although the HAd property apparently serves as an isolate-specific marker, it may be of minor importance immunologically.

The foregoing reference (COGGINS, 1968b) is of particular interest because it is the first time that successful neutralization of ASF virus has been claimed. There is some reluctance to call this true neutralization, for the antiserum must be present in the assay cultures throughout the test period (COGGINS, personal communication). An inhibitory substance might be expected to behave in this manner. However, the specificity of the reaction is more indicative of antibody. In view of the exhaustive efforts of others to demonstrate neutralizing antibodies in swine refractory to challenge inoculation with ASF virus (DE BOER, 1967b; DE BOER et al., 1969), additional information forthcoming on this subject is eagerly awaited.

Some serums from surviving or chronically infected pigs will react with antigens present in infected cell cultures (MALMQUIST, 1963) or certain tissues of acutely infected pigs (COGGINS and HEUSCHELE, 1966; BOULANGER et al., 1967b) to produce precipitin bands in the AGDP test. The number of bands formed depends on the serum used and the source and concentration of the antigen. Isolate-specificity is not apparent. However, some of the antigens responsible for the formation of precipitin bands have been separated by isoelectric precipitation (STONE and HESS, 1965). One of these appears to be isolate-specific. Aside from being a specific isolate marker, the immunological significance of this antigen is not known. Antigens common to all of the isolates appear to be present in much larger amounts than the isolate-specific material, and they probably account for the high degree of cross-reactivity which renders CF, AGDP, FA and ferritin-conjugated antibody techniques ineffective for detecting type or strain differences among the virus isolates (BOULANGER et al., 1967a, b, c; BREESE et al., 1967). Although the noninfectious antigens are disease specific, they have not as yet been identified as viral substances.

Some of the demonstrable antibodies arising from ASF virus infection may not be directed against the infectious virus particle. However, when infected cells treated with ferritin-conjugated ASF antibody globulin are cut in thin sections and examined with the electron microscope, the tagged globulin is found to be closely associated with the virus particle (BREESE et al., 1967). Like CF, FA, and AGDP, the reaction cannot distinguish one virus isolate from another.

Because of its implications concerning the existence of immunologic types among the ASF virus isolates, an observation not previously reported is presented here for consideration (HESS, unpublished). Five pigs that had survived inoculation with the Hinde isolate which had been passaged 75 times in a line of pig kidney cells (PK_{2a}) were inoculated with the virulent Hinde isolate. Four of the animals survived. After 30 days, two of the pigs were moved to another room and were inoculated with the Lee isolate of ASF virus and survived. The remaining two were given a challenge inoculation of Lisbon 1960 virus. They died within 9 days with acute ASF. The pigs that had survived the Lee virus were after 30 days found to be refractory to the Lisbon 1960 isolate as well. These results were reproducible, and similar results have occasionally been obtained with other supposedly heterologous isolates. Apparently there is an overlapping of antigenic properties among the isolates which allows a progressive broadening of the refractory state in an animal if the isolates are administered in the proper order. If this concept is correct, true immunologic types cannot be said to exist.

If the obscure immunology of ASF is ever to be understood, the complex antigenic composition of the virus must be resolved.

D. Effects of Physical und Chemical Agents on Infectivity

The stability of the etiological agent of a contagious disease is always a matter of concern and is usually among the first aspects of the disease problem to be investigated. Adhering to this principle, many of the early investigators of ASF devoted considerable time and effort to determining the effects of a variety of environmental factors and physical and chemical agents on the infectivity of the virus (MONTGOMERY, 1921; STEYN, 1932; WALKER, 1933; GEIGER, 1937; DE KOCK et al., 1940). Since they were obliged to use domestic swine in their tests, the studies were seldom of a quantitative nature. This work has been reviewed elsewhere (NEITZ, 1963), and only a few of the more important aspects of it will be mentioned

1A*

here. Otherwise, the present analysis will be concerned with quantitative information that has appeared recently and is more indicative of intrinsic characteristics of the virus.

Heat inactivation studies (PLOWRIGHT and PARKER, 1967) have revealed that at 37°C the virus in a medium containing 25 per cent serum has a half-life of 23 to 24 hours. Without serum the half-life was reduced to 8 hours. At 56°C, a small fraction of virus retained infectivity for more than an hour. Progeny of this fraction had a profile of thermal stability similar to the original test virus, thus indicating the absence of a genetic basis for the greater resistance of the fraction. Infectivity was completely destroyed in 20 minutes at 60°C. Divalent cations had no effect on thermal stability. In pig blood held at 4°C, the virus was very stable over periods up to 18 months. At −70°C, virus in pig spleen retained its original infectivity titer for at least 2 years. There was a progressive and marked loss of infectivity during storage at −20°C. In two years, titers were reduced by 3 to 4 $\log_{10}$ units. Others have likewise detected a residuum of infectivity after 1 hour at 56°C (COGGINS, 1966) and it is amply apparent that the routine serum inactivation procedure (56°C for 30 minutes) is not adequate when dealing with ASF virus.

The virus is stable over a remarkably broad range of pH (PLOWRIGHT and PARKER, 1967) with persistence of infectivity in alkaline environments being especially notable. Preparations free of serum retained some infectivity as long as 21 hours at pH 13.4. In the presence of 25 per cent serum, the survival time at the same pH was extended to 7 days. In serum-free medium, inactivation was rapid when the pH was below 3.9. One isolate retained infectivity for 4 hours at pH 2.7 and for 2 hours at pH 1.9.

Trypsin, ethylenediaminetetraacetate (EDTA), ultrasonic waves, and alternate freezing and thawing as commonly applied in virus research methods have little or no deleterious effect on infectivity (COGGINS, 1966). Inactivation by 0.05 per cent β-propiolactone, acetylethyleneimine, or glycidaldehyde is achieved in 60 minutes at 37°C without impairing CF activity or the ability to stimulate the production of CF and precipitating antibodies in pigs (STONE and HESS, 1967).

In blood plasma at 25°C, the virus resisted 3 hours' exposure to the direct rays of the sun. However, an ultraviolet radiation dose of 1.5×10^5 erg inactivated the virus in films of plasma in 60 minutes (KOVALENKO et al., 1964).

When it was found that the virus did not survive during centrifugation in a density gradient of cesium chloride, tests were made to determine its sensitivity to salt. Virus suspensions in sodium chloride solutions graduated in concentration from physiologic (0.146 M) to 1.82 M were held at 4°C for 12 hours and then titrated in pig leukocyte cultures and tested for CF activity. Two or 3 $\log_{10}$ units of infectivity were lost in solutions having sodium chloride concentrations greater than 1.0 M (HESS and STONE, unpublished). The CF activity was unaltered. The ions responsible for inactivation have not been determined.

As stated previously, ASF virus is readily inactivated by lipid solvents and pancreatic lipase, but nucleases and a variety of proteolytic enzymes have no effect on its infectivity (HESS and STONE, unpublished). Its ability to survive in putrefying blood (MONTGOMERY, 1921; STEYN, 1932; GEIGER, 1937) is no doubt a reflection of this resistance to the action of enzymes as well as its ability to withstand extreme pH levels.

The prolonged stability of the virus in blood, excretions, and offal (MONT-GOMERY, 1921; KOVALENKO et al., 1965) is especially noteworthy because of its bearing on the establishment of effective sanitary procedures and regulations.

The persistence of infectivity over such a wide range of physico-chemical environments is unusual, and the knowledge of this is of considerable practical value. However, it is obvious that the stability of ASF virus is greatly affected by the composition of the medium in which it is suspended, and it is therefore difficult to deduce intrinsic properties of the virus particle from most of the data thus far compiled. At this point it is hardly advisable to use inactivation data obtained under one set of conditions to predict what will happen under different conditions.

V. Cultivation in Cell Cultures

A. Host-cell Range

Without previous adaptation, isolates of ASF virus may be readily propagated in cultures of leukocytes from swine bone marrow or buffy coat (MALMQUIST and HAY, 1960). Primary cultures prepared from other swine tissues may initially support virus growth at a low level (PLOWRIGHT and FERRIS, 1956—1957; MANSO RIBEIRO, 1961; MALMQUIST, 1962; GREIG et al., 1967) but the virus either disappears after a few passages or a prolonged period of adaptation is required before substantial virus production and CPE occurs with regularity.

The virus may also be cultivated in a variety of stable cell strains, but, here again, a period of adaptation is required before substantial virus production accompanied by CPE is achieved. Stable lines of pig kidney cells have been most frequently used (MALMQUIST, 1962; SANCHEZ BOTIJA, 1962; 1963b; HESS et al., 1965; RUIZ GONZALVO et al., 1966) and the procedures applied to bring about adaptation have varied. In some instances, cell cultures inoculated directly with blood or tissue suspensions from infected swine or with virus propagated in swine buffy coat cultures have been maintained with occasional fluid changes for long periods of time before CPE occurred and subpassages were made (MALMQUIST, 1962). It was found that frequent fluid changes or dispersion of infected cells with trypsin enhanced the adaptation process (HESS et al., 1965). It also appeared that adaptation of the virus to a pig kidney cell line was more readily initiated following preliminary passage in chicken embryo cell cultures. One or two preliminary passages in mixed cultures of swine leukocytes and a line of swine kidney cells appeared to enhance adaptation of virus to the cell line (RUIZ GONZALVO et al., 1966).

Cell lines originating from species other than porcine have also been used to propagate ASF virus. Again, adaptation was required. A strain of the Hinde isolate adapted to a line of PK_{2a} cells was, after additional adaptation, readily propagated in lines of ovine and bovine kidney cells (MALMQUIST, 1962). The Hinde and Uganda isolates of ASF virus after 75 and 21 passages, respectively, in PK_{2a} cells could be cultivated without further adaptation in lamb testicular cells that were established in continuous cultures (HESS et al., 1963).

The Tengani isolate has been produced in large quantities (STONE and HESS, 1967; BREESE et al., 1967) in a stable line of baby hamster kidney (BHK) cells (MACPHERSON and STOKER, 1962). Passage series of Tengani virus in BHK cells have been initiated directly from infected swine spleen or with virus that was passaged 10, 26, or 45 times in swine leukocyte cultures. As it was passaged serially in leukocyte cultures, the virus became progressively more adaptable to BHK cells (HESS, unpublished).

A line of African green monkey kidney (AGMK) cells has been used in studying the synthesis of ASF virus (VIGÁRIO et al., 1967). Although replication of viral DNA and synthesis of some or all of the antigens took place, no infectious virus or HAd were demonstrated. Recently, the VERO line of AGMK cells (YASUMURA and KAWKITA, 1963) has been used to propagate an ASF virus isolated in Italy and the Tengani isolate from Malawi (HESS, unpublished). In both instances, the virus passage series in VERO cells were initiated by inoculation with suspensions of infected swine spleen. After two passages, CPE was evident, and virus titers of the order of 10^7 hemadsorbing units (HAd_{50}) per ml were regularly obtained thereafter. Adaptation was thus achieved in little more than two weeks.

Among the various isolates of ASF virus that have been adapted to cell cultures, at least two, Hinde (MALMQUIST, 1962) and Uganda (HESS et al., 1965) have been induced to form plaques in PK cell strains (PARKER and PLOWRIGHT, 1968). Although the method is presently limited to viruses well adapted to cell cultures, it is an important advance and should prove extremely useful as a research tool.

Because adaptation of the virus is not required, swine buffy coat and bone marrow cell cultures continue to be the only reliable in vitro systems for isolation and assay of ASF virus from the field. However, the fragile nature of these cultures and failure of the cells to multiply and form confluent sheets preclude their use in certain research procedures. Perhaps a stable cell strain exists that is capable of responding rapidly and visibly to field isolates of the virus. The aforementioned rapid adaptation of two isolates to the VERO strain of AGMK cells should encourage testing of other available cell strains regardless of their species origin.

B. Virus Reproductive Cycle in Cell Cultures

Growth curves for ASF virus in swine buffy coat cultures and swine kidney cell lines (PK_{2a} and PK_{13}) have been determined (BREESE and DE BOER, 1966; COGGINS, 1966; PLOWRIGHT et al., 1966). The reproductive cycles are essentially the same in both cell systems except that the onset of CPE and the release of the virus from the cells is considerably slower in the PK cell lines. During the first few hours the virus titers drop below the input level. Virus production then proceeds logarithmically for the next 12 hours or so, and the peak is reached between 24 to 48 hours. Throughout this period in both cell systems, the level of cell-associated virus exceeds that of the supernatant virus. In the buffy coat system, CPE is complete by the third or fourth day. The level of the supernatant virus then begins to exceed that of the cell-associated virus and both begin to decrease slowly during the remaining period of observation. Virus growth cycles in PK cell systems may vary somewhat depending on the cell line used and the degree of adaptation of the virus. Cytopathic changes are first detectable on the third or fourth day and are well advanced or complete by the sixth day. Even then, the cell-associated virus may continue to be at a higher level than the supernatant virus.

C. Replication and Cytopathogenesis in Cell Cultures

1. Light Microscopy

When describing the sequence of changes that take place in cells infected with ASF virus, it is necessary to consider swine leukocyte cultures separately. The large phagocytic mononuclear cells which are the main elements involved in virus replication in these cultures are especially susceptible to infection. In them the entire cycle from infection through virus release and lysis of the cells is more rapid than in other cell systems. The monocytes do not multiply in culture, and except for the occasional formation of syncytia they remain separated from one another. The erythrocytes in the cultures begin to adsorb on the monocytes within 10 hours after infection. Hemadsorption usually precedes cellular changes. After 12 to 18 hours, infected cells begin to show karyorrhexis, and with special staining (MOULTON and COGGINS, 1968) degeneration of the nucleolus is clearly apparent. At about the same time, intracytoplasmic inclusion bodies appear (HAAG and LARENAUDIE, 1965; MOULTON and COGGINS, 1968a). They usually occur as complete or incomplete rings, or sometimes they appear as crescents, solid bodies, or clusters of granules. They are readily seen in Giemsa-stained preparations and have a color similar to the nuclear chromatin. There is seldom more than one inclusion in a cell. In older cultures, syncytia that have formed may be infected. In this instance, the inclusion is usually centrally located and the nuclei are distributed around the periphery of the giant cell. During the period from 20 to 48 hours after infection CPE reaches a peak and progresses to completion. Nuclei become irregular in shape or folded. The cytoplasm is swollen and vacuolated and the inclusions stain more intensely. The cells lyse, contract, and finally detach from the glass. In the final stages, the inclusion bodies are difficult or impossible to discern because of the intense basophilic staining of the contracted cells.

In PK cells (SANCHEZ BOTIJA, 1963b; MOULTON and COGGINS, 1968a) karyorrhexis begins about 48 hours after infection and inclusion bodies appear about the same time. Inclusions are found less frequently in PK cells than in the infected monocytes, but several may occur in a single cell. They are usually somewhat smaller but stain more intensely. They vary in shape and ring forms are not as prevalent. In the advanced stages of infection (after 80 hours or more) cells become contracted or dendritic and finally detach from the glass and lyse. This usually occurs in focal areas and holes are left in the cell sheet.

The inclusion bodies in both cell systems react positively for DNA with the Feulgen and acridine orange stains, and they stain specifically for viral antigen with FA (HEUSCHELE et al., 1966). When infected cell cultures are inoculated with ^{3}H-labeled nucleic acid precursors (VIGÁRIO et al., 1967; MOULTON and COGGINS, 1968a) and subjected to autoradiography, thymidine-^{3}H is incorporated in the cytoplasm at sites of inclusion bodies. It is therefore assumed that the inclusions are sites of viral synthesis.

2. Electron Microscopy

Cultures of a stable line of swine kidney cells were inoculated with ASF virus and harvested at various times during the virus reproductive cycle. Thin sections were prepared and examined by electron microscopy (BREESE and DE BOER,

1966). Although the actual entry of virus into the cell was not seen, sections made immediately after the initial adsorption period showed mature particles lying just inside the cell membrane. Replication starts soon after entry of the virus, and the entire assembly of virus particles appears to take place in the cytoplasm of the host cell. At 24 hours, rather discrete areas of virus formation have appeared, and in them, particles in all the various stages of development are seen. Few particles are seen in the intercellular spaces. After 48 hours, there are rather orderly arrays of ribosome-like bodies about the peripheries of the developing virus particles. These bodies usually remain with the virus throughout its residence in the cell but are not associated with the virion after it has left the cell. As the particles mature, they appear to move in a random fashion from the site of replication to the cytoplasmic membrane. The virion emerges from the cell by budding, and during the process, apparently acquires an outer coat composed of material from the cytoplasmic membrane. As is to be expected from the growth curve, virus is regularly found in the intercellular spaces after 48 hours. Virus replication in the cytoplasm and exit of mature particles through the cell membrane continues until at 96 hours the cell cytoplasm has been almost entirely replaced by viral structures and debris. At this point, the cellular membrane is usually disrupted and both complete and incomplete virus particles are released.

As mentioned previously hydroxyurea (HU) suppresses the production of ASF virus in cell cultures (MOULTON and COGGINS, 1968a). The inhibitory effect is apparent in the morphogenesis of the virus and has been visualized and studied by electron microscopy (BREESE and DE BOER, 1969). In the normal course of replication of the ASF virus particle, it appears that the multilayered outer shell with its distinctive hexagonal shape is assembled before the central DNA core becomes visible. Although particles in all stages of development are seen in sites of virus replication, the vast majority of particles that move to and bud out through the cytoplasmic membrane are complete in structure. If HU (10^{-2} or 10^{-3} M) is added to the culture medium shortly after the cells have been infected, the virus reproductive cycle proceeds as usual with the exception that the DNA core is apparently absent in nearly all of the particles formed. Sites of replication develop and enlarge. Virus particles lacking visible cores move to and exit through the cell membrane and are found in the intercellular spaces. Cytopathic changes occur in the cells, but the infectivity titer is reduced by as much as 4 $\log_{10}$ units. There is little or no reduction in the level of CF antigen produced.

Suppression of the synthesis of viral DNA by HU has been shown with other viruses (MARGARETTEN et al., 1966; ROSENKRANZ et al., 1966; ZAMBERNARD, 1967; LEVY et al., 1968). As might be expected, HU also effects the formation of certain viral antigens. For example, HU inhibits the formation of the structural antigen (V) of adenovirus in KB cells but has little effect on the synthesis of the virus-specific nonstructural antigens (T-antigens) that are produced early in the lytic cycle of adenovirus-infected cells (LEVY et al., 1968). Synthesis of the DNA core of the frog virus, FV3, is inhibited by HU. Although some capsid formation does occur, the incomplete particles apparently do not bud out of the cells (ZAMBERNARD, 1967).

Some of the antigens produced in ASF virus-infected cells may be neither virus nor structural elements of virus. If inhibition of the synthesis of viral DNA is the only effect that HU has on the reproductive cycle of ASF virus, the reagent is of little value in distinguishing between the structural and nonstructural antigens. However, as more is learned about the effects of HU on the formation of other viruses and their antigens, the unique properties of ASF virus may be better understood. At any rate, the reproductive cycle of the virus must be examined more thoroughly, for it is likely to reveal some of the factors that account for the unusual aspects of the immunology and pathogenesis of ASF.

VI. Interaction with Organisms

A. Host Range

Natural infections with ASF virus appear to be confined to porcine species. In Africa, the virus has been recovered from the wart hog (*Phacochoerus* sp.), bush pig (*Potamochoerus* sp.), and giant forest hog (*Hylochoerus* sp.) (STEYN, 1932; DETRAY, 1963; HEUSCHELE and COGGINS, 1965a). Although they serve as a reservoir of the virus, the wild swine of Africa apparently tolerate the infection without suffering ill effects. This is true of experimental as well as natural infections. Wart hogs and bush pigs inoculated with ASF virus (MONTGOMERY, 1921; WALKER, 1933; DETRAY, 1957b; DETRAY, 1963) failed to show clinical signs of disease but usually developed viremia which in one instance persisted for at least 59 days after inoculation. The mode of transmission of the virus among these species and from them to domestic swine is not well understood (DETRAY, 1957b). However, once established in domestic swine, the virus usually gives rise to a highly contagious, acute febrile disease characterized by a short course, high mortality, and gross lesions that closely resemble those of acute hog cholera.

The European wild boar *(S. scrofa ferus)* is susceptible to ASF and may acquire the disease through contact with affected animals (POLO JOVER and SANCHEZ BOTIJA, 1961). The response to infection is like that of domestic swine, and the lesions produced are similar (RAVAIOLI et al., 1967).

The virus of ASF was apparently isolated in Africa from a hippopotamus (DETRAY, 1963) and a porcupine and hyena (COX, 1963). These findings have not been substantiated by additional isolations (COX, 1963; STONE and HEUSCHELE, 1965) nor have efforts been made to experimentally infect these species.

There have been repeated efforts to propagate ASF virus in animals other than swine (MONTGOMERY, 1921; STEYN, 1928; WALKER. 1929; DE KOCK et al., 1940; MALMQUIST, 1957; DE TRAY, 1963; KOVALENKO et al., 1965). The objectives have been (1) to find a suitable and inexpensive laboratory animal; (2) to determine if species other than porcine might be capable of harboring the virus in nature or on the farm; and (3) to find hosts in which the virus might undergo modification. Cattle, horses, sheep, goats, dogs, cats, guinea pigs, rabbits, hedgehogs, hamsters, rats, mice, and various fowl were among the species tested. Although the first two objectives were not achieved, virus propagation was demonstrated in rabbits and goats and there was some success in modifying the agent in these species. After varying numbers of alternating passages in rabbits and swine (NEITZ and ALEXANDER, cited by MACINTOSH, 1952; MENDES and DASKALOS, 1955; BUGYAKI, 1955; LEITE VELHO, 1956; KOVALENKO et al., 1965) it has been possible to adapt the virus to rabbits and produce signs of the disease in these animals. In one instance, the virus appeared to be unaltered in virulence after 85 passages in rabbits (LEITE VELHO, 1956). Others reported substantial attenuation after 100 passages in rabbits (MENDES, 1962). Another attenuated lapinized strain of ASF virus recovered its initial virulence when passaged a number of times in pigs (SANCHEZ BOTIJA, 1962).

Russian investigators (KOVALENKO et al., 1965) have shown that kids 4 to 5 months old could be infected with ASF virus by intraperitoneal inoculation of infected blood. The animals developed symptoms in 6 to 25 days and one kid died after 36 days. Virus was found in the blood 6 days after infection but was no longer present after 30 days. It was present in the spleen after 36 days but not after 70 days. The disease was characterized by hyperthermia, diarrhea, severe emaciation and by lesions in the reticuloendothelial system. The virus was passaged 19 times in kids and appeared to adapt progressively to these animals causing damage to the reticuloendothelial system and accumulating in the spleen.

Although it has not been possible to infect fowl, there has been some success in propagating the virus in embryonated chicken eggs. Virus that had previously been through two alternating pig-rabbit passages followed by 4 consecutive rabbit passages and a pig passage was used to inoculate 8-day-embryonated eggs. The yolk sacs were inoculated, and incubation was at $33°C$. Most of the embryos died 6 or 7 days later (MACINTOSH, 1952). Several intervening passages in swine were required to maintain the virus through 90 passages in eggs (HENNING, 1956). Other attempts to propagate the virus in eggs without intervening animal passages were, for the most part, unsuccessful (MALMQUIST, 1957, cited by DETRAY, 1963). Various routes of inoculation were used, but the virus did not survive beyond the third passage.

Under experimental conditions, efforts to demonstrate contact transmission of ASF virus among wart hogs or from wart hogs to domestic swine usually failed (MONTGOMERY, 1921; WALKER, 1933; DETRAY, 1957 b). It was therefore suspected that arthropods might be responsible for such transmissions in nature. Thus far, certain argasid ticks have been found capable of harboring and subsequently transmitting the virus to domestic swine. In Spain, the virus was recovered from the tick, Ornithodoros erraticus, found in piggeries where ASF outbreaks had occurred (SANCHEZ BOTIJA, 1963 a). These ticks were able to transmit the virus as long as 6 to 12 months after engorgement on ASF-infected animals (SANCHEZ BOTIJA, personal communication cited by HEUSCHELE and COGGINS, 1965 b). In Africa, another argasid tick, Ornithodoros moubata was shown to be capable of transmitting ASF among domestic swine (HEUSCHELE and COGGINS, 1965 b). Transmission was achieved with both adult and nymphal ticks fed sequentially on infected and susceptible swine. Recently, Ornithodoros moubata collected from animal burrows in Tanzania were found to be infected with ASF virus (PLOWRIGHT et al., 1969). The incidence of infection among wart hogs in the area was quite high, and there were no domestic swine within about 100 miles of the area. It could be safely assumed that the ticks had become infected by feeding on wart hogs or possibly other wild animal species that had inhabited the burrows. The virus titers of positive tick pools ranged from $10^{4.2}$ to $10^{7.0}$ HAd_{50}. Since these titers were considerably in excess of the virus levels found in the blood of naturally infected wart hogs, the authors suggest that the titers may be indicative of virus multiplication in the tick. Transovarial infection in the tick has not yet been demonstrated.

B. Pathogenesis in Domestic Swine

Although the disease readily spreads among domestic swine by direct contact, there is uncertainty concerning the route of infection. It is commonly assumed that the virus present in the excretions and secretions of acutely infected animals is transmitted to other animals by nuzzling or ingestion and that primary invasion occurs in the upper respiratory or alimentary tracts (SCOTT, 1965a). On the basis of this assumption, peracute infections produced by instillation of highly virulent strains of ASF virus into the oral or nasal cavities of domestic swine are believed to closely approximate natural infection. Quantitative studies have been made on the sequential development of infections initiated in this manner. Despite marked differences in certain details, the overall findings reported by the various investigators were essentially the same. Whether the virus was inoculated intranasally or into the oral cavity, invasion usually occurred in the upper respiratory tract and spread rapidly to lymph nodes in the cephalic region. In an experiment in which animals weighing 60—80 pounds were inoculated intranasally, initial infection was detected in the tonsils and mandibular lymph nodes at 1-day post-inoculation (DPI) (HEUSCHELE, 1967). In another study (PLOWRIGHT et al., 1968) initial infection usually occurred in the retropharyngeal mucosa and rapidly spread to the retropharyngeal nodes. There was little indication that the tonsils or the nasal or alimentary mucosae were involved during the first 24 hours. Although the animals used in the second study were somewhat smaller (45—55 pounds), the virus isolate and method of exposure were similar in both studies. There is no readily apparent explanation for the differences observed.

From the primary sites of infection in the upper respiratory tract and the adjacent lymph nodes, the virus spread apparently via the lymph ducts and the blood stream to practically all tissues of the body. In one instance, virus was found in circulating leukocytes at 1-DPI (HEUSCHELE, 1967). However, generalized infection was usually demonstrable after 3-DPI. The onset of pyrexia also occurred about that time or within the next 24 hours. The lymphoid tissues involved in the primary infection continued to harbor large quantities of virus throughout the course of the disease. As the infection became generalized, high concentrations of virus appeared in the spleen, bone marrow, liver, and lungs, and these tissues were considered to be the main secondary sites of virus multiplication. Since viremia was usually very pronounced, the virus levels found in many tissues were thought to be due only to the quantities of blood present in them. It was earlier suggested (MAURER et al., 1958) that ASF virus was produced mainly in cells of the reticuloendothelial system since the most severe and significant histopathologic changes were observed in those cells. The results of the quantitative studies of the infection appear to support this belief, for highest virus concentrations were invariably found in tissues having large components of reticuloendothelial cells.

The sequential development of the infection in newborn pigs following instillation of the virus into the oral cavity proceeded as in the older animals but at a more rapid pace (COLGROVE et al., 1969). The tonsils were usually first to become infected and were considered to be the most frequent site of initial entry of the virus. Viremia was demonstrated as early as 8 hours after inoculation, and generalization was well advanced at 30 hours. Whereas the FA technique was not entirely satisfactory for locating ASF viral antigens in tissues of mature swine (HEUSCHELE et al., 1966), it was found that specific fluorescence could be demonstrated regularly in tissue of acutely infected newborn pigs (COLGROVE et al., 1969). It was therefore possible to detect the specific cells involved in the disease process. In lymphatic tissues, antigen was first apparent in the reticular cells and macrophages. In later stages lymphocytes fluoresced. In liver, hepatic cells and mononuclear cells in sinusoids were infected. Septal cells and free macrophages in the lungs were involved. Antigen was detected in megakaryocytes and blast cells in bone marrow and in monocytes in the blood. Late in the infection, viral antigen was found in the endothelium and tunica media of vessels in a number of tissues. In one instance, specific cytoplasmic fluorescence was seen in several epithelial cells exfoliating from the surface of the tonsils. For the most part, the virus showed a definite predilection for cells of the reticuloendothelial system, and in tissues where specific fluorescence was seen, reticular cells, monocytes, and macrophages were the cells usually involved.

The subsequent involvement of the endothelium and tunica media of the blood vessels is consistent with the vascular necrosis and hemorrhages that occur in the terminal stages of ASF and supports an earlier contention (MAURER et al., 1958) that the vascular lesions are due to the direct effect of the virus.

While infection usually developed in the manner described, there was evidence that invasion of the virus by alternate routes sometimes occurred. In one animal, virus was first isolated from the lungs, bronchial mucosa, and bronchial lymph nodes (PLOWRIGHT et al., 1968). The virus had apparently entered through the lower respiratory tract. Occasionally, primary infection was found in the mesenteric lymph nodes of newborn pigs indicating that the virus might have entered via the small intestine (COLGROVE et al., 1969).

Determinations of virus levels in various components of blood from infected animals gave conflicting results and led to differences of opinion concerning the importance of circulating leukocytes in the spread of infection. In one study (HEUSCHELE, 1967) virus was found in the leukocyte fraction as early as 1-DPI although it was not detected in the whole blood or other fractions until 3-DPI. Throughout the first 4 days of the infection, the highest virus titers were consistently found in the leukocyte fraction. It was concluded that infected leukocytes entering the blood stream from infected lymph nodes were instrumental in spreading the virus to other tissues. Again, PLOWRIGHT and his coworkers found that 90 per cent of the circulating virus was associated with the cellular components, but most of it was in the erythrocyte fraction. They further demonstrated in vitro adsorption of ASF virus on normal swine erythrocytes. Intact leukocytes were thought to contribute little to the viremia. However, viral antigen has been demonstrated by the FA technique in leukocytes from the blood of infected newborn pigs (COLGROVE et al., 1969). Specific fluorescence was first seen 48 hours after inoculation and involved only a few cells. It increased thereafter, and frequently involved large numbers of leukocytes in every miscroscopic field examined. Monocytes were most commonly affected, and the fluorescence was associated

with discrete cytoplasmic inclusions. These inclusions were also apparent in leukocytes treated with Giemsa stain. Specific fluorescence was also occasionally seen
in polymorphonuclear leukocytes and a few lymphocytes. It appears likely that
circulating leukocytes may be substantially involved in the spread of infection
in the newborn pig at least.

It should be noted that the HAd phenomenon may occur spontaneously in
leukocyte cultures prepared from the blood of an acutely infected animal. At
times the reaction is very rapid, and though it has not been definitely proven,
there is reason to believe that it may actually occur *in vivo*. At any rate, infected
leukocytes with erythrocytes adhering to their surfaces are likely to be sedimented
with the erythrocyte fraction when the blood components are being separated.
This possibility should be considered when trying to determine the distribution
of ASF virus among the blood fractions.

While it may be concluded that the reticuloendothelial system is the main
target of the virus, there are some differences of opinion concerning the identity
of the cells most commonly involved. Karyorrhexis of lymphocytes has been described as one of the outstanding changes occurring in lymphoid tissues (STEYN,
1928; DE KOCK et al., 1940; MAURER et al., 1958; MANSO RIBEIRO and ROSA
AZEVEDO, 1961; POLO JOVER and SANCHEZ BOTIJA, 1961; KOVALENKO et al.,
1965). Others have indicated that monocytes and macrophage-type cells contained
the viral antigen and degenerated in acute ASF (BOULANGER et al., 1967c; MOUL-
TON and COGGINS, 1968b; COLGROVE et al., 1969). The lymphocytes were often
the last cells to become involved.

Despite the existing areas of disagreement, the overall description of the development of the acute infection in domestic swine appears to be quite complete,
and in general, it is consistent with the clinical signs and the gross and micro-
scopic lesions that are characteristic of the most severe form of the disease. However, little is known concerning the development of the infection in the wart hog
or other wild species, nor have systematic studies been made of the sequential
development of the subacute and chronic forms of ASF in domestic swine.

In areas where ASF has become enzootic in domestic swine, its character has
changed from a peracute disease with mortality approaching 100 per cent to
a disease of lesser mortality with an increased incidence of acute, subacute, and
chronic infections (SANCHEZ BOTIJA and POLO JOVER, 1964; SCOTT, 1965a). It
is often impossible on the basis of clinical signs and gross lesions to distinguish
these forms of ASF from classical swine fever. Of even greater concern is the fact
that carriers have become increasingly important in the maintenance and spread
of the disease in domestic swine. This poses a number of questions that are likely
to be answered only through studying all aspects of the development and persistence of the chronic or latent infection as well as the mechanisms involved in
activating such infections to the extent that transmission may occur.

C. Clinical Manifestations and Pathology in Domestic Swine

Since the clinical manifestations and pathology of ASF have been reviewed
a number of times (NEITZ, 1963; DETRAY, 1963; GIERLØFF, 1963; SCOTT,
1965a,b; LUCAS et al., 1967), only brief descriptions along with an updated
bibliography are presented here.

When describing the clinical and pathologic features of ASF in domestic swine, the responses are usually categorized as peracute, acute, subacute, and chronic. Inapparent infections also occur. Incubation periods measured from the time of exposure to the onset of fever vary with the virus strain, dose, and method of exposure. Following natural or contact exposure, it varies from 5 to 15 days (MONTGOMERY, 1921; WALKER, 1933; LEITE VELHO, 1957; POLO JOVER and SANCHEZ BOTIJA, 1961; DETRAY, 1963). When virus is introduced parenterally, the incubation period may be only 1 day but is usually from 2 to 5 days (MONTGOMERY, 1921; STEYN, 1928; MAURER et al., 1958; DETRAY, 1963). Even with strains modified by passage in cell cultures, the onset of fever if it occurs at all usually appears within the first 15 days following inoculation. In peracute cases, death is often the first indication of the disease, and occasionally it occurs without any obvious gross lesions appearing. Usually definite clinical signs may be observed. There is an abrupt and usually severe thermal response which may persist for 3 or 4 days. During this period the total leukocyte count may fall to about 40 per cent of normal (DETRAY and SCOTT, 1957). Otherwise, the affected animals continue to appear quite normal until the temperature begins to fall. They then stop eating and lie huddled together. If forced to rise and move, they exhibit weakness and incoordination. Within 24 to 48 hours, they are moribund. The pulse and respiration are accelerated and often cyanotic areas appear on the extremities. Vomiting, diarrhea which is occasionally tinged with blood, and mucopurulent conjunctival and nasal discharges are other signs sometimes encountered. Death usually occurs by the seventh day after the onset of fever. The lesions of acute ASF have been described in detail (MONTGOMERY, 1921; STEYN, 1928; WALKER, 1933; GEIGER, 1937; DE KOCK et al., 1940; MAURER et al., 1958; MANSO RIBEIRO and ROSA AZEVEDO, 1961; POLO JOVER and SANCHEZ BOTIJA, 1961; KOVALENKO et al., 1965; NUNES PETISCA, 1965a). As noted in the section on pathogenesis, the virus acts almost exclusively on reticuloendothelial tissues. This is clearly reflected in the histopathology of acute ASF. Severe degenerative changes are seen in lymphoid tissues and in the walls of arterioles and capillaries. In turn, gross lesions which are entirely the consequences of this vascular damage are edema, hemorrhage, occlusions, infarction, and necrosis. There is usually an excess of pericardial, pleural, and peritoneal fluids. Hemorrhages may occur in nearly every organ. The lymph nodes, in particular, are involved and in some instances may resemble blood clots. The spleen is usually red or purple in color and may be severely engorged and enlarged. Congestion and hemorrhage often occur throughout the alimentary tract. The lungs are usually edematous. Epicardial and endocardial hemorrhages are common. The kidneys are often studded with petechiae. In fact, every organ and tissue may show some changes that are attributable to vascular damage.

Before ASF became established as an enzootic disease in domestic swine, subacute and chronic infections were only occasionally encountered, and descriptions were necessarily limited (DE KOCK et al., 1940; DETRAY, 1957a). As the disease spread in Portugal and Spain, there were increased opportunities to observe the less acute forms. However, the use of cell culture-attenuated virus strains as vaccines soon made extensive studies of the chronic disease not only possible but urgently necessary (MANSO RIBEIRO et al., 1963; SANCHEZ BOTIJA,

1963b; Nunes Petisca, 1965b; Moulton and Coggins, 1968b). The chronic
disease observed prior to this was usually in the occasional animal that had
somehow survived after displaying the typical clinical signs of an acute infection
with fully virulent virus. The onset of infection with an attenuated virus may be
marked by only a slight febrile reaction, and the clinical signs of chronic infection
may appear only after some stress has occurred or after exposure to virulent virus.
In either instance, the chronic lesions that develop are similar. Pericarditis, pneumonia, hyperplasia of lymph nodes, and arthritis are the common lesions. Large
cutaneous ulcerations may also occur.

D. Immunity

Swine that have survived primary infection or have been infected with
attenuated strains of ASF virus are often refractory to challenge with the fully
virulent homologous virus. Antibodies readily demonstrable by CF, precipitin
tests, and the HAdI reaction (Malmquist and Hay, 1960; Cowan, 1961; 1963;
Coggins and Heuschele, 1966; Boulanger et al., 1967a, b; Stone et al., 1968)
are usually present in the serums of such animals. However, virus is often con-
comitantly present. Such serums may occasionally have some protective capacity,
for a significant number of animals have survived lethal doses of virus when these
serums have been administered simultaneously (Walker, 1933; DeTray, 1957a).
Nevertheless, practically all efforts to demonstrate virus neutralizing antibodies
have failed (De Boer, 1967b; De Boer et al., 1969), and the only reported
exception to this (Coggins, 1968b) remains to be confirmed. Persistent infection
(DeTray, 1957a; Beveridge, 1963) production of interferon (Malmquist,
1963), and immune tolerance (De Boer, 1967b) have been suggested as possible
mechanisms responsible for the development and maintenance of the refractory
state. All explanations advanced thus far remain hypothetical, and the immunology
of ASF continues to be obscure.

The difficulties encountered in attempting to develop immunizing agents
have only added to the obscurity. All attempts to produce protective antibodies
by administering antigens rendered noninfectious by a variety of physical and
chemical treatments have failed. Such treatments included heat (Montgomery,
1921) Lugol's solution, toluol, formalin (Walker, 1933) crystal violet as used
to produce hog cholera vaccines (De Kock et al., 1940; Mendes, 1953—1954;
DeTray, 1957a; Manso Ribeiro et al., 1958), β-propiolactone (DeTray, 1963;
Stone and Hess, 1967), acetylethyleneimine, and glycidaldehyde (Stone and
Hess, 1967). Antigens treated with some of these agents were capable of stimulating the production of CF and precipitin antibodies, but even when administered in adjuvants, none afforded protection against virus challenge (Stone
and Hess, 1967).

By serial passage in cell cultures, a number of ASF isolates have been sufficiently modified to produce nonfatal infections in domestic swine (Malmquist,
1963; Manso Ribeiro et al., 1963; Sanchez Botija, 1963b; Hess et al., 1965;
Coggins et al., 1968). These animals often have a high level of CF and precipitin
antibodies in their serums and do not develop the usual acute, fatal infection
when their immunity is challenged with homologous virulent virus. Apparently
the attenuated strain must retain some virulence in order to have any protective

value. Such a virus may produce only subclinical infection in healthy animals maintained under ideal conditions of nutrition and sanitation, and these animals may tolerate very large doses of the fully virulent homologous virus. Yet when an attenuated virus of this type was used in a large scale vaccination program (MANSO RIBEIRO et al., 1963) 128,684 animals out of about 550,000 that had received the vaccine developed postvaccinal reactions among which were deaths, pneumonia, locomotor disturbances, skin ulcers, abortions, and disturbances of lactation. Under such conditions inapparent carriers were probably also present. These disturbing sequelae were believed to have resulted from using attenuated virus in the midst of an epizootic of fully virulent ASF. Others who have experimented with live virus vaccines (SANCHEZ BOTIJA, 1963c) have indicated that even without subsequent exposure to virulent ASF virus, a large portion of the vaccinated animals develop chronic infections and mortality eventually may reach 10—50 per cent. A large number of healthy carriers may be produced and remain free of trouble for a long time, but most of them finally die of an acute episode or more often of a chronic pneumonia. The final mortality figures appear to be related to the degree of virulence retained by the strain, the sensitivity of the particular lot of animals tested, and conditions of stress imposed on the inoculated animals. It has been shown experimentally that swine vaccinated with attenuated ASF virus and stressed with foot-and-mouth disease, rinderpest, or hog cholera virus are less able to survive challenge inoculation with virulent ASF virus than those not stressed (DELAY and SHERMAN, 1965).

Obviously, much remains to be learned concerning the immunology of ASF. Under ideal conditions, live attenuated vaccines protect against only a single virus strain, and under adverse conditions in the field, they may actually give rise to chronic and inapparent infections. These should be reasons enough to concentrate more effort on learning the basic immunologic principles involved rather than merely continuing the empirical search for a satisfactory vaccine.

E. Virus Modification in Domestic Swine

Its capacity for change is indeed one of the outstanding properties of ASF virus. Since it is a factor to be considered in practically all phases of research on this disease agent, it has already been mentioned in several places in this review. The change pointed out in each instance was one of decreased virulence for domestic swine, and it came about during passages in cell cultures, embryonated chicken eggs, rabbits, and goats. The changes occurred under controlled experimental conditions and in some instances have been repeated several times. On the other hand, it has been stated a number of times that the virus has undergone modification during the process of becoming established as an enzootic disease agent in domestic swine. Although the present reviewer has accepted this as a likely possibility, it is only fair to point out that this is one mode of virus modification that has not been confirmed experimentally. In fact, the only recorded test of the possibility resulted in an increase rather than a decrease in virulence (DETRAY, 1963). A virus isolate from a wart hog progressively increased in virulence during 45 serial passages in domestic swine. In an experimental passage series of this kind, many of the selective pressures involved in the natural transmission and spread of the virus are no doubt exluded. However, events that have occurred in areas where the disease has become enzootic in domestic swine do not exclude the possibility that the observed changes in the disease might be due to a large extent to the use of live attenuated vaccines.

African swine fever as an enzootic disease of domestic swine was first reported in Angola (MENDES and DASKALOS, 1955). An increase in subacute and chronic infections was soon noted and was attributed to modification of the virus through continuous association with domestic swine (LEITE VELHO, 1956). It should be noted that attenuation of ASF virus was experimentally achieved in Angola by alternate passages in rabbits and swine (MENDES and DASKALOS, 1955; MENDES, 1966). There is nothing in the reports of the testing of this virus to indicate that it could have escaped to the general swine population.

In Europe there can be no doubt that the vaccine virus used (see preceding section) had an excellent opportunity to become widely disseminated. While there is ample experimental evidence that the virus may be attenuated by passage in cell cultures, modification of the virus by passage in domestic swine alone cannot be regarded as an established fact.

F. Diagnosis

Since a satisfactory immunizing agent for ASF is not available, rapid detection and elimination of infected and exposed animals is the procedure employed to halt the spread of the disease. The effectiveness of this "stamping out" method depends to a large extent upon the speed with which it is initiated. Rapid diagnosis is therefore essential.

Although there are a number of disease conditions in swine which may duplicate some of the symptoms of ASF (NEITZ, 1963), the main diagnostic problem is in distinguishing the disease from classical swine fever. However, if the epizootiology suggests the possibility of an ASF outbreak in an area, any febrile, hemorrhagic syndrome occurring in swine and especially in swine that have been immunized against hog cholera should be regarded as highly suspicious. Diagnosis of the disease as it usually occurs in Africa is not especially difficult, and a provisional diagnosis based on the history of the outbreak, the clinical signs, and postmortem findings is usually correct. However, in areas where the disease has become enzootic in domestic swine, the resemblance between ASF and classical swine fever is often so pronounced that clinical pathological differentiation is usually impossible. Positive differentiation in any case requires laboratory confirmation which usually consists of isolation and identification of the virus or demonstration of CF, precipitin, and HAdI antibodies. In areas where vaccination has been practiced virus isolation is required.

Spleen, lymph nodes, liver, and blood are the tissues most useful for laboratory examination. Keeping in mind the fact that some of the laboratory tests are of little value when dealing with chronic or inapparent infections, the tests are presented in the order of their proven reliability.

The cross-immunity test is considered to be most definitive (DETRAY, 1963; SANCHEZ BOTIJA and POLO JOVER, 1964; LUCAS et al., 1967). Animals susceptible and animals immune to classical swine fever are inoculated with a suspension of blood and spleen of the affected animal. If reaction occurs in all of the animals, ASF is indicated. If only the susceptible animals sicken, the suspension contains classical swine fever virus (GEIGER, 1937). French investigators emphasize the necessity for using hyperimmune swine (LUCAS et al., 1967). If animals hyperimmunized against classical swine fever are not available, the test may be conducted by simultaneously inoculating one group of swine with hyper-immune anti-hog cholera serum and the tissue suspension. If ASF-immune swine are also available, a reciprocal cross-immunity test may be conducted (DeLAY and CARBREY, 1963). The procedure could strengthen a diagnosis of classical swine fever.

The HAd test (MALMQUIST and HAY, 1960) affords the most convenient and rapid means of detecting and identifying ASF virus, and modified methods of producing the required leukocyte cultures (HESS and DeTRAY, 1960; TUBIASH, 1963) have made the test feasible as a routine diagnostic procedure. Although the test has proven to be of great practical value (SANCHEZ BOTIJA C. and SANCHEZ BOTIJA R., 1965), some experience is necessary if one is to recognize and minimize the deficiencies and anomalies that are sometimes encountered. Tissue samples from chronic cases or carriers that have died from an acute attack may produce CPE but two or three subpassages in leukocyte cultures may be required before HAd occurs. Strains of ASF virus that do not produce HAd have been demonstrated in the laboratory (COGGINS, 1968 b) and could presumably exist in the field. Non-specific HAd has been reported (KORN, 1963) but the experienced worker has no difficulty in recognizing it. While there may be other viruses that affect swine and are capable of producing HAd (DRÄGER et al., 1965) they do not produce diseases that are likely to be confused with ASF.

If a good ASF antiserum is available, CF (COWAN, 1961, 1963; BOULANGER et al., 1967 a) and AGDP (COGGINS and HEUSCHELE, 1966; BOULANGER et al., 1967 b) tests may be used to detect viral antigen in tissue samples. Immunofluores-cence (HEUSCHELE et al., 1966; BOULANGER et al., 1967 c; COLGROVE, 1968) may also be used. These tests are likely to be of value only when applied to tissues from animals with a primary acute infection.

With the aid of a concentrated antigen prepared from ASF virus-infected cell cultures (MALMQUIST, 1963) the CF and AGDP reactions should be of value in detecting ASF antibodies in serums from chronically infected or carrier swine. The HAdI reaction (MALMQUIST, 1963; CARNERO et al., 1967; COGGINS, 1968a) may be of similar value.

G. Epizootiology

It is impossible to discuss much of the research on ASF without touching upon the epizootiology of the disease. The two enzootic cycles in which the virus exists (SCOTT, 1965a, b) give rise to problems that are distinct and separate and make it difficult to deal with ASF as a single disease entity. Therefore, a number of fea-tures of the epizootiology have already been discussed in the present review. The subject has also been presented a number of times in previous reviews (NEITZ, 1963; DeTRAY, 1963; GEIRLØFF, 1963; SCOTT, 1965a, b; LUCAS et al., 1967). The reviews by SCOTT are especially recommended, for he has developed and emphasized the concept of the dual nature of the epizootiology of ASF. The validity of this concept becomes clearly apparent if one compares recent reports from Europe (SANCHEZ BOTIJA and POLO JOVER, 1964; HAAG, 1964; BOLDRINI,

1967) with a recent report of an outbreak of ASF in Kenya (HEUSCHELE *et al.*, 1965).

Many aspects of the transmission of ASF remain obscure. Although recent work has expanded our knowledge of factors involved in the transmission of the acute disease in domestic swine (KOVALENKO *et al.*, 1965), much is still to be learned concerning transmission among wild swine, from wild swine to domestic swine, and from chronically infected domestic swine to other domestic swine. The possible role of arthropod vectors has been indicated (SANCHEZ BOTIJA, 1963a; HEUSCHELE and COGGINS, 1965b; KOVALENKO *et al.*, 1967; PLOWRIGHT *et al.*, 1969), but the full importance of this means of transmission remains to be accessed. The mode of transmission continues to be the weakest point in our knowledge of the epizootiology of ASF.

References

ADLDINGER, H. K., S. S. STONE, W. R. HESS, and H. L. BACHRACH: Extraction of infectious deoxyribonucleic acid from African swine fever virus. Virology **30,** 750—752 (1966).

ALMEIDA, J. D., A. P. WATERSON, and W. PLOWRIGHT: The morphological characteristics of African swine fever virus and its resemblance to Tipula iridescent virus. Arch. ges. Virusforsch. **20,** 392—396 (1967).

ANDREWES, C. H.: Classification of viruses of vertebrates. Advanc. Virus Res. **9,** 271—296 (1962).

Anonymous: Report of the FAO/OIE emergency meeting on African horse sickness and African swine fever held in Paris, France, January 17—20. Bull. Off. int. Epiz. **55,** 75—537 (1961).

BEVERIDGE, W. I. B.: In: Modern Trends in Immunology. I. Chapter 6, Acquired immunity: Viral infections, pp. 130—144. (R. CRUIKSHANK, ed.) Butterworths, Washington, D.C., 1963.

BIRD, F. T.: On the development of the Tipula iridescent virus particle. Canad. J. Microbiol. **8,** 533—534 (1962).

BOLDRINI, G.: La peste swina Africana in Europa. Una situazione di emergenca che si aggrava. Vet. ital. **18,** 238—261 (1967).

BOULANGER, P., G. L. BANNISTER, D. P. GRAY, G. M. RUCKENBAUER, and N. G. WILLIS: African swine fever. II. Detection of the virus in swine tissues by means of the modified direct complement-fixation test. Canad. J. comp. Med. **31,** 7—11 (1967a).

BOULANGER, P., G. L. BANNISTER, D. P. GRAY, G. M. RUCKENBAUER, and N. G. WILLIS: African swine fever. III. The use of agar double-diffusion precipitation test for the detection of the virus in swine tissues. Canad. J. comp. Med. **31,** 12—15 (1967b).

BOULANGER, P., G. L. BANNISTER, A. S. GREIG, D. P. GRAY, G. M. RUCKENBAUER, and N. G. WILLIS: African swine fever. IV. Demonstration of the viral antigen by means of immuno-fluorescence. Canad. J. comp. Med. **31,** 16—23 (1967c).

BREESE, S. S. JR., and C. J. DE BOER: Electron microscope observations of African swine fever virus in tissue culture cells. Virology **28,** 420—428 (1966).

BREESE, S. S. JR., and C. J. DE BOER: Chemical structure of African swine fever virus investigated by electron-microscopy. J. gen. Virol. **1,** 251—252 (1967).

BREESE, S. S. JR., and C. J. DE BOER: Effect of hydroxyurea on the development of African swine fever virus. Amer. J. Path. **55,** 69—77 (1969).

BREESE, S. S. JR., and W. R. HESS: Electron microscopy of African swine fever virus hemadsorption. J. Bact. **92,** 272—274 (1966).

BREESE, S. S. JR., S. S. STONE, C. J. DE BOER, and W. R. HESS: Electron microscopy of the interaction of African swine fever virus with ferritin-conjugated antibody. Virology **31,** 508—513 (1967).

BUGYAKI, L.: La peste porcine au congo belge. Ann. Soc. belge Méd. trop. **35,** 479—490 (1955).

CAME, P. E., and A. H. DARDIRI: Host specificity and serologic disparity of African swine fever virus and amphibian polyhedral cytoplasmic viruses (33504). Proc. Soc. exp. Biol. (N.Y.) **130,** 128—132 (1969).

CARNERO, R., B. LARENAUDIE, F. RUIZ GONSALVO et J. HAAG: Peste porcine africaine. Etudes sur la réaction d'hémadsorption et son inhibition par des anticorps spécifiques. Rec. Méd. vét. **143,** 49—59 (1967).

CHITWOOD, L. A., and E. C. BRACKEN: Replication of herpes simplex virus in a metabolically imbalanced system. Virology **24,** 116—120 (1964).

COGGINS, L.: Growth and certain stability characteristics of African swine fever virus. Amer. J. vet. Res. **27,** 1351—1358 (1966).

COGGINS, L.: A modified hemadsorption-inhibition test for African swine fever virus. Bull. epizoot. Dis. Afr. **16,** 61—64 (1968a).

COGGINS, L.: Segregation of a nonhemadsorbing African swine fever virus in tissue culture. Cornell Vet. **58,** 12—20 (1968b).

COGGINS, L., and W. P. HEUSCHELE: Use of agar diffusion precipitation test in the diagnosis of African swine fever. Amer. J. vet. Res. **27,** 485—488 (1966).

COGGINS, L., J. MOULTON, and G. COLGROVE: Studies with Hinde attenuated African swine fever virus. Cornell Vet. **58,** 525—540 (1968).

COLGROVE, G.: Immunofluorescence and inclusion bodies in circulating leukocytes of pigs infected with African swine fever virus. Bull. epizoot. Dis. Afr. **16,** 341—343 (1968).

COLGROVE, G., E. O. HAELTERMAN, and L. COGGINS: Pathogenesis of African swine fever virus in young pigs. Amer. J. vet. Res. **30,** 1343—1359 (1969).

COWAN, K. M.: Immunological studies on African swine fever virus. I. Elimination of the procomplementary activity of swine serum with formalin. J. Immunol. **86,** 465—470 (1961).

COWAN, K. M.: Immunologic studies on African swine fever virus. II. Enhancing effect of normal bovine serum on the complement-fixation reaction. Amer. J. vet. Res. **24,** 756—761 (1963).

COX, B. F.: African swine fever. Bull. epizoot. Dis. Afr. **11,** 147—148 (1963).

DE BOER, C. J.: Antibody studies in animals infected with African swine fever virus (ASFV). Fed. Proc. **26,** 482 (1257) (1967a).

DE BOER, C. J.: Studies to determine neutralizing antibody in sera from animals recovered from African swine fever and laboratory animals inoculated with African swine fever virus with adjuvants. Arch. ges. Virusforsch. **20,** 164—179 (1967b).

DE BOER, C. J., W. R. HESS, and A. H. DARDIRI: Studies to determine the presence of neutralizing antibody in sera and kidneys from swine recovered from African swine fever. Arch. ges. Virusforsch. **27,** 44—54 (1969).

DE KOCK, G., E. M. ROBINSON, and J. J. G. KEPPEL: Swine fever in South Africa (East African swine fever). Onderstepoort J. **14,** 31—93 (1940).

DELAY, P. D., and E. A. CARBREY: Experimentally induced hog cholera in pigs immunized with African swine fever virus. Proc. U.S. Livestock Sanit. Ass. **67,** 170—176 (1963).

DELAY, P. D., and E. C. SHARMAN: The effect of stressor viruses on pigs inoculated with attenuated African swine fever virus. Bull. Off. int. Epiz. **63,** 733—749 (1965).

DETRAY, D. E.: Persistence of viremia and immunity in African swine fever. Amer. J. vet. Res. **18,** 811—816 (1957a).

DETRAY, D. E.: African swine fever in wart hogs (Phacochoerus aethiopicus). J. Amer. vet. med. Ass. **130,** 537—540 (1957b).

DETRAY, D. E.: African swine fever. Advanc. vet. Sci. **8,** 299—333 (1963).

DETRAY, D. E., and G. R. SCOTT: The effect of hyperimmune hog cholera serum on the virus of African swine fever. J. Amer. vet. med. Ass. **126,** 313—314 (1955).

DETRAY, D. E., and G. R. SCOTT: Blood changes in swine with African swine fever. Amer. J. vet. Res. **18,** 484—490 (1957).

DRÄGER, K., S. KAMPHANS und D. WEIGAND: Zur Frage der Spezifität des Hämadsorptionstestes bei der afrikanischen Schweinepest. Tierärztl. Umschau **20**, 1—4 (1965).

DUC-NGUYEN, H.: Hemadsorption of mumps virus examined by light and electron microscopy. J. Virol. **2**, 494—506 (1968).

GEIGER, W.: Virusschweinepest und afrikanische Virusseuche der Schweine. Thesis, Hannover (1937).

GIERLØFF, B. C. H.: Europaeisk og afrikansk svinepest. En oversigt. II. Afrikansk svinepest. Nord. Vet.-Med. **15**, 365—394 (1963).

GREIG, A. S., P. BOULANGER, and G. L. BANNISTER: African swine fever. IV. Cultivation of the virus in primary pig kidney cells. Canad. J. comp. Med. **31**, 24—31 (1967).

HAAG, J.: The evolution of African swine fever in Spain. Encyc. Vet. Period. **21**, 168—171 (1964).

HAAG, J., et B. LARENAUDIE: Peste porcine africaine. L'effet cytopathogène du virus en culture leucocytaire. Bull. Off. int. Epiz. **63**, 191—198 (1965).

HAAG, J., B. LARENAUDIE et F. RUIZ GONZALVO: Peste porcine africaine. Action de la 5-iodo-2'-desoxyuridine sur la culture du virus *in vitro*. Bull. Off. int. Epiz. **63**, 717—722 (1965).

HAAG, J., A. LUCAS, B. LARENAUDIE, F. RUIZ GONZALVO et R. CARNERO: Peste porcine africaine. Recherches sur la taille et la morphologie du virus. Rec. Méd. vét. **142**, 801—808 (1966).

HAMMOND, R. A., and D. E. DeTRAY: A recent case of African swine fever in Kenya, East Africa. J. Amer. vet. med. Ass. **126**, 389—391 (1955).

HENNING, M. W.: Animal diseases in South Africa. 3rd ed. Central New Agency, Ltd., South Africa, pp. 869, 871, 874, and 889 (1956).

HESS, W. R., B. F. COX, W. P. HEUSCHELE, and S. S. STONE: Propagation and modification of African swine fever virus in cell cultures. Amer. J. vet. Res. **26**, 141—146 (1965).

HESS, W. R., and D. E. DeTRAY: The use of leukocyte cultures for diagnosing African swine fever (ASF). Bull. epizoot. Dis. Afr. **8**, 317—320 (1960).

HESS, W. R., H. J. MAY, and R. E. PATTY: Serial cultures of lamb testicular cells and their use in virus studies. Amer. J. vet. Res. **24**, 59—64 (1963).

HEUSCHELE, W. P.: Studies on the pathogenesis of African swine fever. I. Quantitative studies on the sequential development of virus in pig tissues. Arch. ges. Virusforsch. **21**, 349—356 (1967).

HEUSCHELE, W. P., and L. COGGINS: Isolation of African swine fever virus from a giant forest hog. Bull. epizoot. Dis. Afr. **13**, 255—256 (1965a).

HEUSCHELE, W. P., and L. COGGINS: Studies on the transmission of African swine fever virus by arthropods. Proc. U.S. Livestock Sanit. Ass. **69**, 94—100 (1965b).

HEUSCHELE, W. P., L. COGGINS, and S. S. STONE: Fluorescent antibody studies on African swine fever. Amer. J. vet. Res. **27**, 477—484 (1966).

HEUSCHELE, W. P., S. S. STONE, and L. COGGINS: Observations on the epizootiology of African swine fever. Bull. epizoot. Dis. Afr. **13**, 157—160 (1965).

KORN, G.: Über die afrikanische Schweinepest und die Spezifität des Hämadsorptionstestes zu ihrer Diagnose. Mschr. Tierheilk. **15**, 225—232 (1963).

KOVALENKO, J. R., M. A. SIDOROV, and L. G. BURBA: Viability of African swine fever virus in external environment. Vestnik Sel'skokhoz. Nauki **9**, 62—65 (1964) (in Russian).

KOVALENKO, J. R., M. A. SIDOROV, and L. G. BURBA: Experimental investigations on African swine fever. Bull. Off. int. Epiz. **63** bis, 169—189 (1965).

KOVALENKO, J. R., M. A. SIDOROV, and L. G. BURBA: II. Pasture ticks and haematopinus as possible reservoirs and vectors of African swine fever. Trudy Vses. Inst. eksp. Vet. **33**, 91—94 (1967) (in Russian).

LARENAUDIE, B., J. HAAG et R. CARNERO: La purification du virus de la peste porcine africaine par le fluorocarbone. Bull. Off. int. Epiz. **63**, 711—716 (1965).

LARENAUDIE, B., J. HAAG et B. LACAZE: Identification en France métropolitaine de la peste porcine africaine ou maladie de Montgomery. Bull. Acad. vét. Fr. **37**, 257—259 (1964).

LARENAUDIE, B., M.-C. TOULIER, J. SANTUCCI et R. CARNERO: Etude en microscopie électronique de l'hémadsorption provoquée par le virus de la peste porcine africaine. Rec. Méd. vét. **143**, 925—935 (1967).

LEITE VELHO, E.: Observations sur la peste porcine en Angola. Bull. Off. int. Epiz. **46**, 335—340 (1956).

LEITE VELHO, E.: La peste porcine africaine. Bull. Off. int. Epiz. **48**, 395—402 (1957).

LEVY, J. A., R. J. HEUBNER, J. KERN, and R. V. GILDEN: High titre T antigen with minimal amounts of structural antigen in adenovirus-infected cells treated with hydroxyurea. Nature (Lond.) **217**, 744—745 (1968).

LUCAS, A., et R. CARNERO: Situation du virus de la peste porcine africaine dans la systématique virale. C. R. Acad. Sci. (Paris) **266**, 1800—1801 (1968).

LUCAS, A., J. HAAG et B. LARENAUDIE: Les procédures du diagnostic de laboratoire utilisées en France a l'égard des pestes porcines. Choix, applications, résultats, enseignements. Bull. Off. int. Epiz. **63**, 723—731 (1965).

LUCAS, A., J. HAAG et B. LARENAUDIE: La peste porcine africaine (Maladie de Montgomery). L'expansion Editeur (1967).

LUNGER, P. D., and P. E. CAME: Cytoplasmic virus associated with Lucké tumor cells. Virology **30**, 116—126 (1966).

MACPHERSON, I., and M. STOKER: Polyoma transformation of hamster cell clones — and investigation of genetic factors affecting cell competence. Virology **16**, 147—151 (1962).

MALMQUIST, W. A.: Propagation, modification and hemadsorption of African swine fever virus in cell cultures. Amer. J. vet. Res. **23**, 241—247 (1962).

MALMQUIST, W. A.: Serologic and immunologic studies with African swine fever virus. Amer. J. vet. Res. **24**, 450—459 (1963).

MALMQUIST, W. A., and D. HAY: Hemadsorption and cytopathic effect produced by African swine fever virus in swine bone marrow and buffy coat cultures. Amer. J. vet. Res. **21**, 104—108 (1960).

MANSO RIBEIRO, J.: Communication à l'Office International des Epizooties, Session générale. Bull. Off. int. Epiz. **56**, 1212—1214 (1961).

MANSO RIBEIRO, J.: Communication à l'Office International des Epizooties, Session générale, Bull. Off. int. Epiz. **58**, 1031—1040 (1962).

MANSO RIBEIRO, J., J. L. NUNES PETISCA, F. LOPES FRAZAO et M. SOBRAL: Vaccination contre la peste porcine africaine. Bull. Off. int. Epiz. **60**, 921—937 (1963).

MANSO RIBEIRO, J., et J. A. ROSA AZEVEDO: La peste porcine africaine au Portugal. Bull. Off. int. Epiz. **55**, 88—106 (1961).

MANSO RIBEIRO, J. J. A. ROSA AZEVEDO, M. J. O. TEIXEIRA, M. C. BRACO FORTE, A. M. RODRIGUES RIBEIRO, F. OLIVEIRA E. NORONHA, C. GRAVE PEREIRA et J. DIAS VIGARIO: Peste porcine provoquée par une souche différente (Souche L) de la souche classique. Bull. Off. int. Epiz. **50**, 516—534 (1958).

MARGARETTEN, W., C. MORGAN, H. S. ROSENKRANZ, and H. M. ROSE: The effect of hydroxyurea on virus development. I. Electron microscopy study of the effect on the development of bacteriophage T4. J. Bact. **91**, 823—833 (1966).

MAURER, F. D., R. A. GRIESEMER, and T. C. JONES: The pathology of African swine fever — a comparison with hog cholera. Amer. J. vet. Res. **19**, 517—539 (1958).

MACINTOSH, B. M.: The propagation of African swine fever virus in the embryonated hen's egg. J. S. Afr. vet. med. Ass. **23**, 217—220 (1952).

MENDES, A. M.: Preparacao de una vacina contra la peste suina en Angola. Pecuaria **47**, 56 (1953—1954).

MENDES, A. M.: The lapinization of the virus of African swine fever. Bull. Off. int. Epiz. **58**, 699—705 (1962).

MENDES, A. M.: African swine fever. An. Esc. sup. Med. vet. Lisboa **8**, 199—216 (1966).

MENDES, A. M., y A. M. DE O. DASKALOS: Algunas tentativas para a liporizacao de virus de peste suina em Angola. Rev. Cienc. Vet. Lisbonne **50**, 253—264 (1955).

MONTGOMERY, R. E.: On a form of swine fever occurring in British East Africa (Kenya Colony). J. comp. Path. **34**, 159—191, 243—262 (1921).

MOULTON, J., and L. COGGINS: Synthesis and cytopathogenesis of African swine fever virus in porcine cell cultures. Amer. J. vet. Res. **29**, 219—232 (1968a).

MOULTON, J., and L. COGGINS: Comparison of lesions in acute and chronic African swine fever. Cornell Vet. **58**, 364—388 (1968b).

NEITZ, W. O.: African swine fever. In: FAO. Emerging Diseases of Animals. FAO Agricultural Studies **61**, 1—70 (1963).

NUNES PETISCA, J. L.: Etudes anatomopathologiques et histopathologiques sur la peste porcine africaine (virose L) au Portugal. Bull. Off. int. Epiz. **63** bis, 103—142 (1965a).

NUNES PETISCA, J. L.: Quelques aspects morphologiques des suites de la vaccination contre la peste porcine africaine (virose L) au Portugal. Bull. Off. int. Epiz. **63** bis, 199—237 (1965b).

PARKER, J., and W. PLOWRIGHT: Plaque formation by African swine fever virus. Nature (Lond.) **219**, 524—525 (1968).

PINKERTON, H., C. N. SUN, D. HENSON, and J. NEFF: Human cytomegalovirus: intranuclear virus-synthesizing bodies. Virology **24**, 498—500 (1964).

PLOWRIGHT, W., F. BROWN, and J. PARKER: Evidence for the type of nucleic acid in African swine fever virus. Arch. ges. Virusforsch. **19**, 289—304 (1966).

PLOWRIGHT, W., and R. D. FERRIS: Research in tissue culture: African swine fever. East Afr. vet. Res. Org. An. Rep. p. 28 (1956—1957).

PLOWRIGHT, W., and J. PARKER: The stability of African swine fever virus with particular reference to heat and pH inactivation. Arch. ges. Virusforsch. **21**, 383—402 (1967).

PLOWRIGHT, W., J. PARKER, and M. A. PIERCE: African swine fever virus in ticks (*ornithodoros moubata*, Murray) collected from animal burrows in Tanzania. Nature (Lond.) **221**, 1071—1073 (1969).

PLOWRIGHT, W., J. PARKER, and R. F. STAPLE: The growth of a virulent strain of African swine fever virus in domestic pigs. J. Hyg. (Lond.) **66**, 117—134 (1968).

POLO JOVER, F., y C. SANCHEZ BOTIJA: La peste porcina africana en España. Bull. Off. int. Epiz. **55**, 107—147 (1961).

Proposals and Recommendations of the Provisional Committee for Nomenclature of Viruses (PCNV): Ann. Inst. Pasteur **109**, 625—637 (1965).

RAVAIOLI, L., E. PALLIOLA e A. IOPPOLO: La peste swina Africana dei cinghiali. Nota I: Possibilità d'infezione sperimentale da inoculazione. Vet. ital. **18**, 499—513 (1967).

ROSENKRANZ, H. S., H. M. ROSE, C. MORGAN, and K. C. HSU: The effect of hydroxyurea on virus development. II. Vaccinia virus. Virology **28**, 510—519 (1966).

RUIZ GONZALVO, F., J. HAAG, R. CARNERO et B. LARENAUDIE: Peste porcine africaine. Adaptation d'une souche de virus aux cultures de rein de porc. Rec. Méd. vét. **142**, 1237—1249 (1966).

SANCHEZ BOTIJA, C.: Estudios sobre la peste porcina africana en España. Bull. Off. int. Epiz. **58**, 707—727 (1962).

SANCHEZ BOTIJA, C.: Reservorios del virus de la peste porcina africana. Investigación del virus de la P.P.A. en los artrópodos mediante la prueba de la hemoadsorcion. Bull. Off. int. Epiz. **60**, 895—899 (1963a).

SANCHEZ BOTIJA, C.: Modificación del virus de la peste porcina africana en cultivos celulares. Contribución al conocimiento de la acción patógena y del poder de protección de las estirpes atenuadas. Bull. Off. int. Epiz. **60**, 901—919 (1963b).

SANCHEZ BOTIJA, C.: La peste suina Africana. Zooprofilassi **18**, 587—607 (1963c).

SANCHEZ BOTIJA, C., y F. POLO JOVER: Informe sobre algunos aspectos de la peste porcina africana en España en 1964. Bull. Off. int. Epiz. **62**, 945—952 (1964).

SANCHEZ BOTIJA, C., y R. SANCHEZ BOTIJA: El diagnostico de la peste porcina africana por la prueba de la hemoadsorción (test de Malmquist y Hay). La interferencia del virus de la peste clásica del virus de la peste africana como medio de identificación del virus de la peste clásica en los cultivos de leucocitos. Bull. Off. int. Epiz. **63** biz, 239—251 (1965).

SCOTT, G. R.: The virus of African swine fever and its transmission. Bull. Off. int. Epiz. **63**, 645—677 (1965a).

SCOTT, G. R.: Symposium: The Smallest Stowaways. I. African swine fever. Vet. Rec. **77**, 1412—1427 (1965b).

STEYN, D. G.: Preliminary report on a South African virus disease amongst pigs. S. Afr. Director of Vet. Educ. and Res. 13th and 14th Report, p. 415—428 (1928).

STEYN, D. G.: East African virus disease in pigs. Union of South Africa, Director of Vet. Serv. and Anim. Ind. 18th Rep., pp. 99—109 (1932).

STONE, S. S., P. D. DELAY, and E. C. SHARMAN: The antibody response in pigs inoculated with attenuated African swine fever virus. Canad. J. comp. Med. **32**, 455—460 (1968).

STONE, S. S., and W. R. HESS: Separation of virus and soluble noninfectious antigens in African swine fever virus by isoelectric precipitation. Virology **26**, 622—629 (1965).

STONE, S. S., and W. R. HESS: Antibody response to inactivated preparations of African swine fever virus in pigs. Amer. J. vet. Res. **28**, 475—481 (1967).

STONE, S. S., and W. P. HEUSCHELE: The role of the hippopotamus in the epizootiology of African swine fever. (A survey of the incidence of African swine fever in hippopotami in Queen Elizabeth Park, Uganda.) Bull epizoot. Dis. Afr. **13**, 23—28 (1965).

TUBIASH, H. J.: Quantity production of leukocyte cultures for use in hemadsorption tests with African swine fever. Amer. J. vet. Res. **24**, 381—384 (1963).

VIGÁRIO, J. D., M. E. RELVAS, F. P. FERRAZ, J. M. RIBEIRO, and C. G. PEREIRA: Identification and localization of genetic material of African swine fever virus by autoradiography. Virology **33**, 173—175 (1967).

WALKER, J.: Memorandum on research on East African swine fever immunization in Kenya. Proc. Pan-African Conf., Pretoria, pp. 1—13 (1929).

WALKER, J.: East African Swine Fever. Baillière, Tindall and Cox, London, p. 139 (1933). Thesis: Vet. Fac. Univ. Zurich, Switzerland.

WATRACH, A. M.: Intranuclear filaments associated with infectious laryngotracheitis virus. Virology **18**, 324—327 (1962).

WEISSENBERG, R.: Fifty years of research on the lymphocystis disease of fishes (1914—1964). Ann. N.Y. Acad. Sci. **126**, 362—374 (1965).

YASUMURA, Y., and Y. KAWKITA: Studies on SV 40 in tissue culture. Nippon Rinsho. **21**, 1201—1219 (1963).

ZAMBERNARD, J.: The effect of p-fluorophenylalanine and hydroxyurea on the replication of a frog kidney virus. J. Cell Biol. **35**, 191A—192A (1967).

ZWILLENBERG, L. O., and K. WOLF: Ultrastructure of lymphocystis virus. J. Virol. **2**, 393—399 (1968).

ZWILLENBERG, H. H. L., und L. O. ZWILLENBERG: Über den Erythrocytenabbau in der Forellenmilz unter besonderer Berücksichtigung der Erythrocytenfeinstruktur. Z. Zellforsch. **60**, 313—324 (1963).

Addendum

During the interim between the writing and publishing of this review, a number of reports on African swine fever have appeared. Additional studies on ASF virus infection in *Ornithodoros moubata porcinus* are of particular interest (PLOWRIGHT *et al.*, 1970). It is now definitely established that virus multiplication and transovarial infection occur in this species of *Argasid* ticks. The importance of this arthropod in the maintenance and spread of ASF virus in Africa is evident.

Levels of a number of serum enzymes in swine have been found to be substantially altered during ASF virus infection (COMPAGNUCCI et al., 1969). Effects of ASF virus infection on certain of the host's enzyme systems are also being studied at the cellular level (POLATNICK and HESS, 1970). Although work has only begun in this area, it is already apparent that much information on the disease process may be derived from studying the host's enzyme systems.

References

COMPAGNUCCI, M., F. MARTONE e A. VACCARO: Ricerche sul comportamento di alcuni enzimi (GOT, GPT, Al., LDH, LAP, SDH, Fac totale e FAI) nel siero di suini con peste suina Africana. Vet. ital. **20,** 385—402 (1969).

PLOWRIGHT, W., C. T. PERRY, M. A. PEIRCE, and J. PARKER: Experimental infection of the Argasid tick, *Ornithodoros moubata porcinus*, with African swine fever virus. Arch. ges. Virusforsch. **31,** 33—50 (1970).

POLATNICK, J., and W. R. HESS: Altered thymidine kinase activity in cultured cells inoculated with African swine fever virus. Amer. J. vet. Res. **31,** 1609—1613 (1970).

Bluetongue Virus

By

P. G. Howell and **D. W. Verwoerd**

Sections of Virology and Molecular Biology,
Veterinary Research Institute,
Onderstepoort, Republic of South Africa

With 4 Figures

Table of Contents

I. Introduction	37
II. Historical	37
III. Virus Replication in Laboratory Host Systems	38
A. Tissue Culture	38
1. Host Cell Range	38
2. Growth Cycle	39
3. Plaque Formation	40
4. Inhibitors and Interference	40
5. Morphological Aspects of Replication	40
6. Effect of Virus Replication on Cellular Metabolism..........	41
B. Embryonated Chicken Eggs	41
C. Laboratory Animals	43
1. Mice	43
2. Hamsters	44
IV. Properties of the Virion	44
A. Purification	44
B. Morphology	45
C. Physico-chemical Characteristics	47
1. Physical Properties	47
2. Chemical Composition	47
3. Secondary Structure of the Viral Nucleic Acid..............	48
D. Resistance to Physical and Chemical Agents	49
1. Thermal Inactivation	49
2. pH Stability	50
3. Chemical Agents	50

  V. Antigenic Characteristics 50
      A. Serological Reactions 50
          1. Neutralization... 50
          2. Complement Fixation 51
          3. Gel Precipitin Reactions 52
          4. Fluorescent Antibody 53
          5. Haemagglutination 53
      B. Antigenic Variation 53
      C. Distribution of Antigenic Types 55
 VI. Interactions with Mammalian Hosts 56
      A. Pathogenesis 56
      B. Essential Clinical Features 58
      C. Pathology 60
          1. Macroscopic Pathology 60
          2. Histopathology... 61
          3. Clinical Pathology 63
      D. Immunity 63
          1. Immunological Response to Bluetongue Virus 63
          2. Active Immunization 65
      E. Epizootiology.. 66
VII. Classification and Nomenclature 68
References 69
Addendum 74

I. Introduction

Bluetongue may be described as an acute insect borne disease of ruminants, manifested clinically in sheep by a catarrhal inflammation of the mucous membranes of the digestive and respiratory systems and associated with degenerative changes in the skeletal musculature. The profound emaciation and weakness which follow the acute disease are responsible for a protracted convalescence and for serious economic losses due to diminished productivity.

II. Historical

During the early colonisation of Africa, susceptible Merino and other European breeds of sheep were introduced into the Cape, at first by the Dutch East India Company between 1652 and 1785 and again later in 1870. A report of the Cattle and Sheep Diseases Commission (1876) records the appearance of a serious febrile disease amongst these imported sheep in which both morbidity and mortality was high (cited by HENNING, 1949). HUTCHEON (1881) gave this disease the name of "Fever" or "Epizootic Catarrh", in order to distinguish it from other clinical conditions of a similar nature encountered amongst sheep. In the first comprehensive description of this clinical syndrome and its epizootiology HUTCHEON (1902) referred to it as "Malarial Catarrhal Fever of Sheep", a designation which was obviously influenced by the mistaken belief that an intracorpuscular parasite was the primary cause of the disease.

More systematic studies were conducted by SPREULL (1902; 1905), who endeavoured to immunize sheep by the simultaneous inoculation of immune serum and infective blood. Much was added to current knowledge of the epizootiology of the disease at that time and the experimental reproduction of the clinical disease by a cell free filtrate was confirmed.

THEILER (1906) established the filterable nature of the causal agent and considered it to be a virus closely associated with the blood, but not exclusively with the red corpuscles. While practicing the method of immunization suggested by SPREULL, THEILER (1908) reported on the apparent attenuation of a strain of virus after limited serial passage in sheep. This strain was used as a vaccine for nearly 40 years and over 50 million doses were issued. The original method of production, described by ALEXANDER and HAIG (1951), was modified by DU TOIT (1929 b) who also replaced, for a short period, the original strain used by THEILER.

The rapid growth of the sheep breeding industry brought to light the apparent inefficiency of THEILER's vaccine, in so far as it failed to provide adequate immunity in the field. This led NEITZ (1948) to conclude from his *in vivo* studies, that a plurality of virus strains existed in nature. The successful propagation of the virus in the developing chicken embryo provided a suitable host system for the development and production of a polyvalent vaccine incorporating live attenuated strains of virus (ALEXANDER, 1947). Nevertheless, in spite of its susceptibility, the chicken embryo failed to provide the necessary incentive to the investigation of the more fundamental characteristics of the virus.

Following the general pattern in virus research, adaptation of the virus to tissue culture by HAIG, McKERCHER and ALEXANDER (1956) provided a convenient method for the production of sufficient quantities of virus for purification and investigations into the physical properties of the virus. Similarly, the serum-virus neutralization test in cell cultures led to the identification of several specific immunological groups.

During recent years the rapid spread of the disease from Africa to other continents of the world gave further impetus to its study. Previously extensions of the disease occurred at periodic intervals, into the Eastern Mediterranean countries (GAMBLES, 1949; TAMER, 1949; KOMAROV and GOLDSMIT, 1951). This was followed in more recent years by a spread to North America (HARDY and PRICE, 1952; McGOWAN, 1953; BOWNE, LUEDKE, JOCHIM, and FOSTER, 1964), the Iberian Penninsula (MANSO-RIBEIRO, ROSA-AZEVEDO, NORONHA, BRACO FORTE, JR., GRAVE-PEREIRA, and VASCO-FERNANDES, 1957; CAMPANO LOPEZ and SANCHEZ BOTIJA, 1958) and West Pakistan in 1959 (SARWAR, 1962). A bluetongue-like disease which broke out amongst cattle in Japan during the period 1959 to 1960 has been described by OMORI (1961), INABA, ISHII, and OMORI (1966), and ISHITANI (1967). A virus isolated during the course of this epizootic appears, on the basis of certain biological and physico-chemical properties, to resemble bluetongue virus very closely (MIYAMOTO, TAKEHARA, NOMURA, SAME-JIMA, and NAKAMURA, 1962—1963). Serological tests, conducted between this virus and various strains of bluetongue, however, have elicited no cross neutralization or complement fixation and the identity of this virus thus remains obscure. Based on clinical evidence the disease has also been reported in India in 1963 [FAO/OIE (1964), SAPRE (1964)].

III. Virus Replication in Laboratory Host Systems

A. Tissue Culture

1. Host Cell Range

The multiplication of 5 strains of egg adapted bluetongue virus in primary monolayer cultures of lamb kidney cells was first described by HAIG, McKERCHER, and ALEXANDER (1956). These authors furthermore observed that the cytopathic effects of the virus strains could be inhibited by homologous immune sheep serum and pointed out the possible usefulness of this technique for conducting *in vitro* serum-virus neutralization tests in this system. Two attempts to propagate unmodified bluetongue virus in sheep kidney cells, using acute phase serum as inoculum, were unsuccessful and consequently the authors expressed the opinion that cytopathic effects could not be demonstrated on primary isolation of the virulent virus in tissue cultures.

The cell changes observed under low power magnification were recorded by these and other workers. The earliest evidence of virus multiplication and the associated cell destruction may be present as early as 24 hours after infection of the cultures, although an incubation period of 46 to 72 hours is more commonly encountered. At first the cytopathic effects are confined to a few foci of cells which appear enlarged and more refractile. These affected cells give the appearance of becoming swollen to the point of rupture, whereupon they detach from the glass and float free in the nutrient medium. The process of cell destruction progresses rapidly and ultimately involves all the cells of the monolayer. Similar observations were made by PINI, COACKLEY, and OHDER (1966 b).

FERNANDES (1959 a) reported the successful propagation in primary lamb kidney monolayer cultures of both egg adapted and virulent strains of virus, the latter having been obtained from the blood of a reacting sheep in the acute phase of the disease. Further passage of the virus was accomplished without difficulty in a line of human amnion cells, but the cytopathic changes in these cells were considered to be somewhat different to those seen in the cultures of lamb kidney cells. In a comparative study of the susceptibility of various cell lines using cytopathogenesis as an indication of virus multiplication, it was found that monolayer cultures of human amnion, Chang Liver, clonal HeLa and HB2, were the most susceptible, whereas cultures of McCoy synovial, Henle's intestine, bovine kidney, NCTCA 2414 clonal human skin and Chang conjunctiva were less susceptible. Two cell lines, one of human lung (HL-S) and another of kitten lung (KL), developed in the presence of tobacco smoke condensate, were not affected morphologically.

In a later report FERNANDES (1959 b) infected explants of 3,960 primary cultures of various tissue from newborn lambs, including kidney cortex and medulla, tongue, nasal mucosa, conjunctiva, muscle, liver and spleen, with 100 $TCID_{50}$ of tissue culture adapted virus. Complete cell destruction occurred within 6 days without apparent differences in the susceptibility of the various tissues, except that the fibroblasts appeared to be more susceptible than the epithelial-like cell types.

Various observations indicate that strains of bluetongue virus, particularly those which have undergone preliminary adaptation to fertile hen's eggs or passage in tissue culture, may be propagated in other cell types, including bovine foetal kidney (GIRARD, RUCKERBAUER, GRAY, BANNISTER, and BOULANGER, 1967), calf adrenal, calf testis and certain stable cell lines such as BHK-21 and NCTC929 strain L mouse fibroblast.

2. Growth Cycle

The appearance and progress of cytopathic changes is consistent with an increase in the titre of infective virus. In a study of the growth cycle of a type 3 strain of tissue culture adapted virus in primary lamb kidney cells, adsorption of the virus was rapid at 37° C and a delay of 18 hours was recorded between the detection of virus within infected cells and the ultimate liberation of the virus into the nutrient medium. During the course of vaccine manufacture in which egg attenuated strains of bluetongue virus are cultured in primary lamb kidney cells, it has been observed that individual strains exhibit a very consistent growth pattern, but differ from one another in their rate of multiplication and the yield of infective virus.

The development of a plaque assay technique enabled HOWELL, VERWOERD, and OELLERMANN (1967) to determine both the rate of adsorption and growth cycle with greater accuracy. Using a type 4 strain of virus it was found that adsorption at pH 7.4 and a temperature of 37° C was approximately exponential during the first 15 minutes, during which period 95% of the virus was absorbed.

The growth curves of a type 10 bluetongue virus in Earles' L-fibroblasts and BHK-21 cells are shown in Fig. 1. A lag phase of approximately 4 hours was found,

after which the plaque titre rose to reach a maximum after 11 to 12 hours incubation. Approximately 20% of the total viral progeny was liberated from the
cells 24 hours after infection.

3. Plaque Formation

In NCTC strain L fibroblast monolayers under 0.5% agarose in nutrient
medium, 16 heterologous tissue culture- and 14 egg-adapted strains of virus
produced plaques of variable size and morphology. Variations in the rate of
plaque development between strains suggested differences in the rate of multiplication in this cell type, while plaque size and plating efficiency was influenced
by the composition and depth of the overlay.

The plaque assay has since replaced other methods for the routine determination of virus concentration and the detection of neutralizing antibody by
plaque inhibition techniques (HOWELL, VERWOERD, and OELLERMANN, 1967).

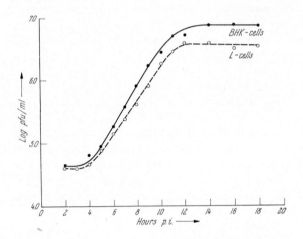

Fig. 1. The growth curve of bluetongue virus in monolayers of
BHK-21 (●———●) and L-cells
(○ – – –○). Titres represent infectious virus liberated into the
medium and determined by means
of a plaque-assay on L-cells

4. Inhibitors and Interference

Replication of bluetongue virus in L and BHK-21 cell lines is not affected
by FUDR or guanidine, but the process is very sensitive to actinomycin D. At
a concentration of 0.1 µg/ml Actinomycin D, the yield of plaque forming units
in BHK cells is only 55% of that produced in the absence of the inhibitor (VER-
WOERD, 1969). Bluetongue virus was found to stimulate interferon formation in
primary mouse cells, but not in the L strain of cells. A yield of approximately
360 units/ml interferon was obtained in the serum of mice 8 hours after infection
with bluetongue virus using the inhibition of ECBO virus plaque formation on
L cells as an indicator system (HUISMANS, V.R.I. Onderstepoort, personal communication). The influence of interferon on the replication of bluetongue virus
has not yet been investigated.

5. Morphological Aspects of Replication

Electron microscopy of the fine structural changes in cells following infection
with bluetongue virus has been reported on by LECATSAS (1968). Adsorption to
and penetration of the virus into the cell was found to occur within the first

5 to 10 minutes, the particle entering the cell by means of a pinocytotic vesicle. The following changes were noticed in the infected cells: First there was the development of dense inclusion bodies, swelling of the endoplasmic reticulum and the appearance of masses of fine filaments in the cytoplasm. Inclusion bodies and bundles of tubular elements also developed in the mitochondria as well as dense bodies containing virus particles. Mature virus was liberated mostly by rupture of the cell membrane and not by budding off. The mature virus particles were shown to be devoid of envelopes.

6. Effect of Virus Replication on Cellular Metabolism

Very little is known regarding the effect of bluetongue virus on the metabolism of cultured cells. There may be some inhibition of both cellular DNA and RNA synthesis. Synthesis of viral RNA commences approximately 3 hours after infection and precedes the detection of infectious progeny virions by approximately 1 hour. A considerable amount of virus-induced RNA synthesis is still found 12 to 14 hours after infection i.e. after the maximal concentration of virus has been reached (HUISMANS, V.R.I. Onderstepoort, personal communication). This phenomenon is also found in reovirus-infected cells (SHATKIN and RADA, 1967).

B. Embryonated Chicken Eggs

The successful propagation of bluetongue virus in fertile hens' eggs was first reported by MASON, COLES, and ALEXANDER (1940). As a result of difficulties experienced in the recovery of virus from infected sheep and subsequent adaptation to growth in fertile hens' eggs, ALEXANDER (1947) investigated the role of the temperature of incubation on the multiplication of the virus in the developing embryo. With the Bekker strain (Type 4) it was found that the infection of 8-day-old embryos by the yolk sac route produced consistently higher yields of virus when incubation was conducted at 32.1°C compared to incubation at higher temperatures. The mortality of embryos incubated at 32.1°C was highest on the 3rd and 4th days after infection and by the 5th day the majority of embryos were dead. Incubation at 35°C resulted in an increased survival time and a reduced yield of virus. The maximal yield of infective virus was obtained when embryos were infected with 500 MID_{50} of virus, incubated at 34°C for 24 hours and then at 32.1°C until death of the embryos on the 3rd or 4th days. ALEXANDER, HAIG, and ADELAAR (1947), working with the "University Farm" (type 9) strain, showed that adaptation was more readily achieved at 33.6°C, but not at 32.1°C, or 38.2°C. After only 3 serial passages at 33.6°C it was possible to continue propagation at either of the two temperatures, but not at 38.2°C. Embryo mortality was similarly found to be more consistent at the lower temperatures and when this was increased to 35°C an increase was noted in the number of survivors. With serial egg to egg passage of the strain at 32.1°C attenuation occurred within 20 passages, whereas at least 100 subcultures were required at an incubation temperature of 35°C. McKERCHER, McGOWAN, and SAITO (1954) similarly reported a more rapid adaptation and attenuation of the American BT8 (type 10) strain of virus when incubation was conducted at 33.5°C as against 36.5°C. This strain was also found to adapt more readily to the chicken embryo when the chorio-allantoic route of inoculation was employed. PRICE and HARDY (1954) reported that they were unable to propagate virulent virus from sheep in eggs at 38°C.

During the isolation of numerous virus strains from field outbreaks in recent years as well as the attenuation of strains representing each of the immunological types in fertile eggs, it has been shown conclusively that a temperature of 33.5°C throughout the period of incubation can be used successfully.

SVEHAG (1963a) studied the growth cycle of the egg-adapted BT8 strain at the 160th passage level. After infection of 7-day-old embryos with 500 LD_{50} via the yolk sac route, 50 to 75% of the virus was adsorbed after 1 hour's incubation at 37°C, whereas less than 50% was adsorbed at 32°C. Similarly the lag phase was shorter at 37°C than at 32°C or 34°C. At the time of peak infective virus production, tenfold more virus was produced at 34°C than at 37°C. At low virus input ratios, a single cycle of virus multiplication was believed to take 36 hours to complete. From these experiments it was shown that a linear relationship could be established between the concentration of virus inoculated and the survival time of the infected embryo.

The growth curves of each attenuated strain used for routine vaccine production, before the introduction of tissue culture, showed a highly consistent growth pattern. It was observed that these growth cycles differed not only between strains of one serological group and another but also between strains of identical origin but passaged independently. Maximum infective virus titres were obtained after 36 to 72 hours incubation at 33.5°C and varied in titre between strains from 10^{-6} LD_{50} to $10^{-8.7}$ LD_{50} per ml. Strains exhibiting the shortest growth cycle consistently produced the highest titres of infective virus. The yolk sac route of inoculation was used for many years and primary isolation and titration of adapted virus was undertaken by this technique. Alternate methods have however been used. GORHAM (1957) described a simple technique for the inoculation of the chorio-allantoic membrane of chicken embryos and VAN ROOYEN and WEISS (1959) drew attention to the advantages of this method over those previously used for the inoculation of bluetongue virus. These workers showed that embryos infected by this "stab" method died more consistently and that the yield of infective virus was generally higher. Embryos infected by limiting dilutions in a titration, died after a shorter incubation period and with greater regularity than embryos infected by the yolk sac route. SVEHAG (1963a) using twofold dilutions of virus, obtained results which indicated that the stab method was slightly more sensitive than the yolk sac route, although irregularities were encountered in the titration of the virus by this method. On the other hand unexpected survivals occurred in the higher virus dilutions that were not seen when the yolk sac route was used.

GOLDSMIT and BARZILAI (1965) studied the susceptibility of 13-day-old embryos to a virulent type 4 strain of bluetongue virus administered by the intravenous route. By comparison with the yolk sac route of inoculation the virus adapted more rapidly with this method and produced 100% mortality by the 3rd passage. At the same time, higher concentrations of infective virus were detected in whole embryo suspensions. Compared with the intravenous route, a thousandfold greater concentration of virus was necessary to establish infection by the yolk sac route.

This intravenous technique should thus prove a great asset in the isolation of virus from samples of low infectivity.

During virus multiplication in embryonated eggs, maximum virus concentrations are reached 6 to 8 hours before death of the embryos as revealed by transillumination. The destructive effect of bluetongue virus on the embryo has been described by MANSO-RIBEIRO and NORONHA (1958). Macroscopically the embryo has a cherry red appearance as a result of extensive haemorrhages, while microscopically the cells of the muscles, liver, kidney, brain and blood vessels show marked degenerative changes.

During the course of the routine examination of numerous field specimens, representing various antigenic types of virus, it has been found that the fertile hens' egg still represents the most susceptible host system for the isolation of virulent virus, when compared with primary cultures of lamb kidney cells (HO-WELL, KÜMM, and BOTHA, in press).

C. Laboratory Animals
1. Mice

KOMAROV and GOLDSMIT (1951) described the isolation of a strain of virus in Israel and claimed that the virus had been successfully adapted to suckling mice.

Quantitative studies of the multiplication of bluetongue virus in mice have been undertaken with various strains. Working with the Cyprus strain (type 3) at the 126th egg passage level, VAN DEN ENDE, LINDER, and KASHULA (1954) showed that preliminary adaptation by the intracerebral route was most successful in suckling mice of 2 to 4 days of age. These workers failed to produce infection in mice older than 12 days. Intracerebral injection of 3 to 4-week-old mice elicited no signs of illness, although there was evidence of limited multiplication and persistence of the virus for at least fourteen serial intracerebral passages. In both suckling and 3 to 4-week-old mice the first evidence of multiplication was found approximately 8 to 12 hours after injection and was considered to be the time taken for a single multiplication cycle of the virus in mouse brain tissue.

SVEHAG (1962) studied the multiplication of the 180th egg passage of the California BT 8 strain in mice. In this study it was shown that the relationship between the age of the mouse and its susceptibility was influenced by the mouse passage level of the virus used. Whereas virus of the 7th mouse passage produced mortality in 1 but not 2-week-old mice, the 53rd passage level of the virus killed mice up to 5 months of age. With increasing age of the mouse there was a marked prolongation of survival time and reduced virus multiplication in the brain tissue. A detailed study of the growth cycle in the brains of 3 to 4-day-old mice revealed a pronounced drop in infectivity 6 hours after inoculation, which was followed by an apparent two phase logarithmic increase in virus concentration.

The symptoms exhibited by suckling mice infected with mouse-adapted strains of virus may be observed from 36 hours post inoculum. At this stage the mice cease suckling, leave the nest and become scattered in the litter. At first they are lethargic but may be stimulated to brief periods of hyperactivity. As the disease progresses, their movements become more incoordinated and prostration develops. Affected mice may be found in a comatose state for a period of 6 to 12 hours before death. Virus concentration appears to increase until the time of death, when titres of between 10^{-6} and 10^{-8} mouse LD_{50} per gram of brain tissue may be obtained. The concentration of virus in the spleen, liver and carcass is very low.

Strains of virus representing all the established antigenic types have been successfully adapted to multiplication in the brains of 3 to 4-day-old mice. The majority of strains were only adapted after one or two preliminary passages in fertile hens' eggs. The type 12 strain required 6 passages in eggs before adaptation to suckling mice was successful. With all the type strains, 100% mortality was obtained after three to four serial passages. After the 5th to 6th passage the mean incubation period was reduced to 3 days. Successful infection of adult or suckling mice with either virulent or mouse- or egg-adapted virus by the intraperitoneal or intranasal route of inoculation has not been reported. Primary isolation of field strains of virus in suckling mice by the intracerebral route has likewise proved unsuccessful. However, it has been reported that infective brain suspensions injected subcutaneously in the neck region of suckling mice, caused nervous symptoms after a prolonged incubation period in about 50% of mice (SVEHAG, 1962).

2. Hamsters

The multiplication of eight strains of mouse- and egg-adapted bluetongue virus in the brains of suckling hamsters was reported by CABASSO, ROBERTS, DOUGLAS, ZORZI, STEBBINS, and COX (1955). The symptoms exhibited by hamsters were similar to those observed in suckling mice. With serial intracerebral passage in hamsters the incubation period was reduced from 4 to 2 days. Hamster brain suspensions however, appeared to yield lower concentrations of virus per gram of tissue compared with suspensions of infective suckling mouse brain. Direct adaptation of chick embryo propagated strains to the brains of suckling hamsters was also possible, although incubation periods were longer than those obtained with mouse-adapted virus. As in the case of the suckling mouse, this host system does not appear to be sufficiently susceptible to unmodified virus to permit its use for the primary isolation of virus. The suckling hamster would appear to be a satisfactory host for the qualitative serum-virus neutralization test, or the preparation of complement-fixing antigens.

IV. Properties of the Virion

A. Purification

Few attempts to purify the bluetongue virus have been reported. In 1948, POLSON used spleen extracts clarified by adsorption onto aluminium hydroxide or by trypsin digestion for his determinations of particle size by ultrafiltration and ultracentrifugation. OWEN and MUNZ (1966) purified material derived from cell cultures by trypsin treatment, differential centrifugation and equilibrium density gradient centrifugation in CsCl. STUDDERT, PANGBORN, and ADDISON

(1966) utilized differential centrifugation as the sole means of purifying their preparations, but mentioned that unsatisfactory results were obtained. These authors, who were primarily interested in electron microscopy, did not determine the yields of infective virus obtained.

A study of the effect of various purification procedures under fully controlled conditions on the infectivity of the virus has been reported by VERWOERD (1969). Two main obstacles were encountered during this investigation. Firstly the virus, though stable in serum and other biological fluids, was found to be extremely unstable after all proteinaceous material had been removed. Secondly the virus exhibited a very strong tendency to adhere to cellular material, a characteristic shared with the reoviruses. Those methods previously devised for the liberation of reoviruses, including freezing and thawing, trypsin digestion, ultrasonication and deoxycholate treatment, were found to be unsuitable for bluetongue virus because of its instability. Stabilization by the addition of proteins and polydextran increased the yields of infective virus but a completely satisfactory answer to the problem has not yet been found.

A purification procedure was eventually adopted in which a concentration step was avoided by extraction of virus from the cellular debris, since about 80% of the virus yield in cell cultures remained cell-bound even after 2 to 3 days. Cells were ruptured osmotically, digested with the aid of chymotrypsin and the cytoplasmic extracts treated with fluorocarbon in the presence of Sephadex G200. This was followed by treatment with Tween 80 and ether and separation of the virus by centrifugation on a sucrose gradient. Final purification could be attained by isopycnic density gradient centrifugation on preformed CsCl gradients, but due to the high salt concentration an excessive loss of virus occurred in this final step.

B. Morphology

In the first electron-micrographs of bluetongue virus to be published, OWEN and MUNZ (1966) described particles showing evidence of an icosahedral shape. Some particles appeared to be enveloped, and had an approximate diameter of 100 mμ in comparison with the naked capsids with an average measurement of 60 mμ. "Empty" capsids were also found and the number of capsomeres were estimated to be 92. Evidence of an outer envelope, possibly derived from proliferation of cytoplasmic membranes, was also presented by BOWNE and JONES (1966) in their study of the virus particles present in salivary glands of *Culicoides variipennis*.

STUDDERT, PANGBORN, and ADDISON (1966) described particles with a diameter of 53 mμ, a hexagonal shape and an internal diameter in empty particles of approximately 40 mμ. They also estimated the capsid to consist of 92 capsomeres, but found no evidence of an envelope. Based on these observations, they suggested a morphological resemblance to reoviruses.

These observations were extended in a recent study (ELS and VERWOERD, 1969). What was previously thought to represent envelopes was shown to be cellular membranes occasionally wrapped around one or more particles. These structures, termed pseudo-envelopes, could be removed by treatment with Tween 80 and ether without loss of infectivity, and are not therefore considered part of the virus.

The criteria for icosahedral symmetry of the hexamer-pentamer type, put forward by CASPAR and KLUG (1962) were met by the demonstration of two neighbouring 5-co-ordinated capsomeres with adjacent 6-co-ordinated units in micrographs of highly purified bluetongue virus of both virulent and attenuated strains.

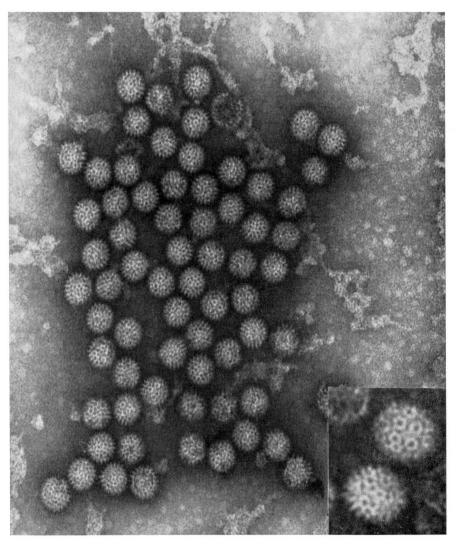

Fig. 2. The ultrastructure of bluetongue virus. Preparations were negatively stained with phosphotungstic acid. Final magnification ×200,000 (inset ×440,000). Micrograph by courtesy of H. J. ELS, unpublished results

From these micrographs a capsomere number of 32 were derived, in contrast to the 92 suggested by previous workers. The high-resolution micrographs presented in Fig. 2 distinctly shows the tubular capsomeres on the surface of the virion and an approximate count made directly, yields a figure of either 32 or

42 of these units. No evidence was found of a double layered capsid as in the case of reovirus.

Evidence was also obtained suggesting that the capsomeres themselves have a hexagonal or pentagonal shape and consist of smaller structural units.

C. Physico-chemical Characteristics

1. Physical Properties

The size of the bluetongue virus was first determined by POLSON (1948), utilizing ultra-filtration and ultra-centrifugation. The particle size of $100-150$ mμ from ultra-filtration data seemed to be confirmed by his ultracentrifugation experiments yielding a figure of $108-133$ mμ. Later reports, based on electron microscopy, demonstrated unequivocally that the diameter of the capsid lies between 50 and 60 mμ (OWEN and MUNZ, 1966; STUDDERT, PANGBORN, and ALLISON, 1966; ELS and VERWOERD, 1969). The fact that the virion is sometimes surrounded by a pseudo-envelope and adheres strongly to cellular material probably introduced this error into the earlier work. This is further born out by the fact that POLSON reported a density of 1.147 gm/cm³ in a sucrose solution, a value later demonstrated to represent the density of virions attached to cellular material (VERWOERD, 1969). The latter author considered the buoyant density of the virus to be 1.38, based on isopycnic density gradient centrifugation data, but considerable difficulty was experienced in obtaining the true value because of the problems encountered in removal of extraneous material during purification of the virus.

Analytical sedimentation studies have not been carried out for the same reason. VERWOERD (1969) reported an approximate sedimentation constant of 653 Svedbergs, determined by the method of POLSON and VAN REGENMORTEL (1961). The biphasic curve obtained in this experiment showed that a considerable percentage of virions in a partly purified virus suspension sediment at a very much lower rate, their lower density being due to adherence of cellular material.

2. Chemical Composition

The first indication that bluetongue virus contains RNA as its genetic material was derived from cytochemical studies using the acridine orange staining procedure (LIVINGSTON and MOORE, 1962). Clearly defined orange-red inclusion bodies were observed in the cytoplasm from 4 hours after infection. Similar results were obtained by WEISS (V. R. I., Onderstepoort, personal communication), with the additional observation that early in the infection cycle these inclusions stain rather heterochromatically, whereas in the later stages the brick-red staining is more pronounced. This phenomenon has also been observed in reoviruses (MAYOR, 1965).

BOWNE and JOCHIM (1967) described RNA-positive bodies in the cytoplasm as well as DNA-positive intranuclear inclusions.

In reovirus infected cells double-stranded RNA is mainly formed during the early stages while single-stranded RNA, considered to act as virus messenger-RNA is detected during the later stages of the replication cycle (PREVEC and GRAHAM, 1966; SHATKIN and RADA, 1967). Similar results have recently been obtained in experiments with bluetongue virus (HUISMANS, V. R. I. Onderstepoort, personal communication).

Chemical analysis of purified bluetongue virus indicated that the virion is composed of $20.0 \pm 1.0\%$ of RNA and $80 \pm 1\%$ of protein. A small amount of phospholipid (1 to 2%), consisting mainly of cholesterol was found, but this is considered to be due to contamination with cellular material (VERWOERD, 1969). The base composition of the RNA (Table 1) was similar to that of reovirus (SHATKIN and SIPE, 1968). The $\frac{A+G}{U+C}$ ratio of 1.004 strongly indicated a double-stranded RNA. All attempts to date to isolate infectious RNA have been unsuccessful.

Table 1. Base Composition of Bluetongue Virus RNA[1]

Preparation	A	U	G	C	$\frac{A+G}{U+C}$	G+C
Bluetongue, unfractionated	31.5	28.4	19.8	20.3	1.05	40.1
Bluetongue, double-stranded	28.3	29.0	21.6	20.8	1.00	42.4
Reovirus[2], unfractionated	29.7	30.5	19.3	20.5	0.96	39.8
Reovirus[3], double-stranded	26.7	25.4	24.2	24.4	1.0	48.6
Reovirus, single-stranded	88.7	9.3	0.9	1.0	8.7	1.9

[1] Expressed as mole percentages (VERWOERD, 1969).
[2] GOMATOS and TAMM (1963).
[3] SHATKIN and SIPE (1968).

3. Secondary Structure of the Viral Nucleic Acid

In order to confirm the apparent double-strandedness of the bluetongue virus genome, RNA was isolated from purified virus and submitted to thermal denaturation and ribonuclease degradation (VERWOERD, 1969). A melting curve typical for double-stranded RNA was obtained, with a Tm of 95°C in SSC-buffer (Fig. 3).

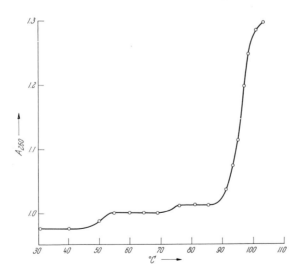

Fig. 3. Thermal denaturation profile of RNA extracted from purified bluetongue virus. Heating was carried out in SSC (0.15 M sodium chloride + 0.15 M sodium citrate)

A consistent double profile was found, indicating contamination of the double strand with an RNA melting at a temperature between 70°C and 80°C. This material could either be cellular contaminants such as t-RNA possessing secondary structure, or a single-stranded virus component such as the adenine-rich 2S molecules found in reovirus (BELLAMY, SHAPIRO, AUGUST, and JOKLIK, 1967; SHATKIN and SIPE, 1968).

Treatment with ribonuclease at a concentration of 2 µg/ml for 30 minutes at 37°C yielded 65% acid-precipitable counts compared to 5% in a control of single-stranded RNA, thus indicating considerable resistance to degradation by this enzyme. It can therefore be concluded that the bluetongue virus genome consists mainly of double-stranded RNA.

Purified virus was also degraded and centrifuged on a sucrose-SDS-urea gradient to obtain more information on the RNA components. The results obtained (Fig. 4) again closely simulate the pattern in reovirus, showing a 2S component, which is probably single-stranded, as well as three double-stranded components of approximately 8S, 10S and 12S (VERWOERD, 1969). It is therefore apparent that the bluetongue and reoviruses are very similar in so far as their nucleic acid is concerned.

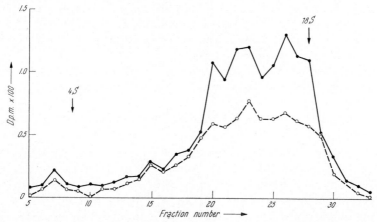

Fig. 4. Sedimentation pattern of RNA from purified, C¹⁴-labelled bluetongue virus in a sucrose-SDS gradient. Virus was disrupted by adding sodium acetate, SDS and urea and directly layered on a SDS-containing 10−30% sucrose gradient and centrifuged for 9 hours at 40,000 r.p.m. RNase treatment was for 30 minutes at 37°C at an enzyme concentration of 1 µg/ml. (●————●) Before, (○— —○) after RNase treatment

D. Resistance to Physical and Chemical Agents

1. Thermal Inactivation

Somewhat conflicting results regarding the thermal stability of bluetongue virus have been published. The demonstration of viable virus in serum stored at room temperature for 25 years indicated a marked thermostability (NEITZ, 1948). Slow freezing at −10° or −20°C was reported to have a deleterious effect on the infectivity of the virus (ALEXANDER, 1947; KIPPS, 1958; HOWELL, VERWOERD, and OELLERMANN, 1967). SVEHAG (1963b) studied the thermal inactivation at pH 7.0 under various conditions and confirmed the marked thermostability, but did not observe the deleterious effect of slow freezing. His thermal inactivation curves suggested first order kinetics with two components at 37°C, 46°C and 56°C. The two-component curves were interpreted to indicate phenotypically determined heterogeneity of the virus population. Thermodynamic data indicated protein inactivation at higher temperatures (46—56°C) and ribonucleic acid inactivation within a lower temperature range (37—46°C). These authors all used unpurified virus preparations containing extraneous proteins. Howell, Verwoerd, and Oellermann (1967) studied the stability of purified virus preparations at temperatures both below and above 4°C and concluded that the virus is extremly unstable particularly at higher temperatures, when all extraneous protein is removed. Thermostability could be enhanced by the addition of 1% albumin, serum, peptone or other protein-derived substances.

2. pH Stability

The stability of bluetongue virus in a pH range between 5.5 and 8.0 has been studied by Owen (1964). At 4°C a marked loss of infectivity occurred below pH 6.5, whereas the virus remained stable between pH 6.5 and 8.0. It was also shown that the persistence of virus in carcass meat was dependent on the post-mortal pH changes. Complete inactivation occurred when the pH dropped below 6.3. Svehag, Leendertsen, and Gorham (1966) found a narrow zone of stability between pH 6.0 and 8.0. Inactivation curves for pH values between 7.2 and 9.0, at different salt concentrations indicated maximum stability at pH 9.0 and low ionic concentrations (Verwoerd, 1969).

The marked sensitivity to acid constitutes an important difference between bluetongue and reoviruses, the latter being considered acid-resistant.

3. Chemical Agents

Sensitivity to ether and sodium deoxycholate is one of the common characteristics of most arboviruses (Andrewes, 1964). Because it is transmitted by arthropod vectors, the bluetongue virus has been regarded as an arbovirus until it was found to be resistant to both these substances (Howell, 1963; Andrewes, 1964; Studdert, 1965; Svehag, Leendertsen, and Gorham, 1966). The degree of resistance is dependent on the presence of extraneous proteins since purified virus was found to be sensitive to deoxycholate. However, inactivation of purified virus is slow when compared to that of the arboviruses and does not therefore invalidate the argument against bluetongue virus belonging to this group.

The effectiveness of five chemicals frequently used as disinfectants was evaluated by McCrory, Foster, and Bay (1959). Wescodyne was found to be the most effective at concentrations above 750 p.p.m., inactivating the virus in undiluted suspensions of infected chicken embryos within 4 to 6 minutes.

V. Antigenic Characteristics

A. Serological Reactions

1. Neutralization

Serum-virus neutralization is the serological test most commonly used for antibody determination and the typing of bluetongue virus strains.

A number of host systems have been used for this technique with varying success. Using suckling mice inoculated by the intracerebral route, Kipps (1958) was able to demonstrate antigenic differences between 6 strains of virus and their antisera in cross neutralization tests. The antigenic specificity of the 16 proto-

type strains has been confirmed in this laboratory in unpublished experiments in
suckling mice, using mouse-adapted strains and convalescent sheep antisera (Ho-
WELL, unpublished). CABASSO, ROBERTS, DOUGLAS, ZORZI, STEBBINS, and COX (1955)
gave a brief description of neutralization tests conducted in suckling hamsters.

ALEXANDER (cited by McKERCHER, McGOWAN, and SAITO, 1954) expressed
the opinion that fertile hens' eggs, injected via the yolk sac route, were unsuitable
for neutralization tests. This was ascribed to the dissociation of the virus antibody
complex brought about by the process of dilution. McKERCHER and co-workers
believed that this problem could be overcome by selecting the chorio-allantoic
membrane route of inoculation, but from their investigations they concluded that
this system was not sufficiently sensitive to detect low antibody concentrations
in convalescent sheep sera, which were nevertheless positive by parallel tests conducted in suckling mice.

This opinion of the value of the fertile hens' egg, as an indicator of virus
neutralization, does not appear to have been shared by other workers. SVEHAG
(1963) used the embryonated egg inoculated by means of the stab method and
via the yolk sac route for his studies on the effect of different contact conditions
on the bluetongue virus-antibody reaction. KLONTZ, SVEHAG, and GORHAM (1962)
similarly used the fertile hen's egg, as a system for establishing the onset, development and persistence of circulating neutralizing antibody in experimentally
infected sheep. GOLDSMIT and BARZILAI (1965) reported that virus was fully
neutralized by homologous serum, when mixtures were inoculated by the yolk
sac and intravenous routes.

The potential value of tissue cultures for neutralization tests was suggested
by HAIG, McKERCHER, and ALEXANDER (1956). Roller tube cultures have subsequently been used by a number of investigators for the quantitative determination of neutralizing antibody or for the detection of antigenic differences amongst
strains (FERNANDES, 1959a; HOWELL, 1960; LIVINGSTON and HARDY, 1964;
JOCHIM, LUEDKE, and BROWNE, 1965).

It is difficult to interpret or compare the results of neutralization tests from
different laboratories, since there has been little uniformity in techniques. Variables have included both serum or virus concentrations, route of infection, dose
and the method of assessing end points. The studies of the virus-antibody reaction
described by SVEHAG (1963a; 1966) should provide a common basis on which
more uniform techniques might be developed. In this study it was shown that by
conventional neutralization tests with limited contact conditions the "Percentage Law" was invalid at low virus doses, whereas with more favourable contact
conditions extending over 24 hours at 37°C the "Percentage Law" became valid
for all virus doses. When reaction mixtures were held under both conventional and extended contact conditions, no reversibility of the virus antibody
reaction was demonstrable by dilution of the reaction mixtures at neutral pH.
Antibody titres were increased up to a hundredfold when the extended contact
conditions were compared with conventional methods.

2. Complement Fixation

The fixation of complement by the bluetongue antibody-antigen complex
was first demonstrated by VAN DEN ENDE, LINDER, and KASCHULA (1954). These

workers used antigens prepared from the brains and cords of infected baby mice by aceton-ether extraction, crude saline extraction, saline extracts clarified by simple centrifugation as well as saline suspensions extracted with equal volumes of ether.

KIPPS (1956) also used suckling mouse brain antigens in the form of acetone-ether extracts and clarified 10% saline suspensions in a series of micro cross-complement fixation tests with 6 strains of bluetongue virus and their homologous antisera. Differences in the reactions between strains were considered to be due to the variables of the extraction procedure. Evidence was presented that the soluble antigen obtained from acetone-ether extracted brains consisted of small particules of 8 mμ whereas crude saline extracts yielded larger particles of varying size, suggestive of aggregates of the 8 mμ particles intermediate in size between the soluble antigen and untreated infective virus. The use of suckling mouse brain as a source of antigen for routine complement fixation tests appears to be favoured by most laboratories.

Tissues and fluids from infected chick embryos have been used with varied success in the preparation of complement fixing antigens. McKERCHER, McGOWAN, and SAITO (1954) used allantoic fluid and the supernatant fluids obtained from centrifuged suspensions of 10% chorio-allantoic membrane. Unsatisfactory results were generally obtained from the antigens of embryonic origin, which proved to be either anticomplementary or otherwise exhibited no antigenic activity after treatment. In this laboratory, antigens consisting of washed saline extracts of infective chorioallantoic membranes have been found to give a reliable indication of the presence of virus.

SHONE, HAIG, and McKERCHER (1956) showed that infective tissue culture fluids could be used as antigens and claimed that little difficulty was experienced with anticomplementary activity. Their antigens showed no immunological specificity and could thus be used to detect the presence of antibodies in sheep sera to either homologous or heterologous strains of virus. The use of the complement fixation test as an aid in the diagnosis and detection of bluetongue antibody has been investigated by ROBERTSON, APPEL, BANNISTER, RUCKERBAUER, and BOULANGER (1965) and BOULANGER, RUCKERBAUER, GRAY, and GIRARD (1967). These authors failed to show any trace of fixation by the direct test with either sheep or calf sera. A modified direct test, in which a normal bovine serum fraction and heated guinea pig serum was added to the complement, gave satisfactory fixation with sera of both species (BOULANGER, 1960).

3. Gel Precipitin Reactions

The application of the agar gel diffusion technique to the detection of precipitating antibody in convalescent sheep antisera was reported by KLONTZ, SVEHAG, and GORHAM (1962). Antigens were prepared from infective suckling mouse brain, chicken embryos and bovine kidney cell cultures. Optimal conditions for the precipitin reaction were obtained in a 1.25% agar base prepared in a phosphate buffer pH 7.2 to 7.4. The reagent cups were spaced 0.5 cm apart and plates were incubated for 116 to 120 hours at 37°C. The lack of correlation between infectivity titres and the concentration of the reactants required for precipitate formation indicated that the precipitating antigen was essentially of a noninfectious nature.

The gel precipitin reaction was shown to be group specific. In this respect an antigenic component common to all strains has similarly been demonstrated by means of the fluorescent antibody technique (PINI, COACKLEY and OHDER, 1966b).

4. Fluorescent Antibody

This technique has been used by RUCKERBAUER, GRAY, GIRARD, BANNISTER, and BOULANGER (1967) for the detection of bluetongue virus in bovine foetal kidney cell cultures inoculated with blood and tissues from experimentally infected animals.

5. Haemagglutination

To date all attempts to demonstrate haemagglutination by conventional techniques, including the use of extracted mouse brain antigens as described for arboviruses, have been unsuccessful. Haemadsorption in tissue cultures with cells of various species has also failed.

B. Antigenic Variation

In an attempt to explain the continued and increasing number of vaccinal failures encountered amongst flocks of immunized sheep, NEITZ (1948) carried out a series of cross-protection tests in sheep with 10 strains of virus, which had been recovered from both cattle, sheep and *Culicoides* over a period of 40 years. It was established that each strain produced a solid and durable immunity against itself, but only a variable degree of protection to challenge by heterologous strains, thus discrediting the suggestion that the immunity produced by THEILER's monovalent vaccine was of a transient nature. A plurality of antigenically different strains of virus was thus established. There appeared to be an antigenic component common to all the strains investigated and an additional unknown number of different specific antigenic characteristics. These experimental results, as well as those of subsequent years, revealed that this *in vivo* technique was unsuitable for the classification of strains into groups on the basis of similar antigenic structure. This is supported by the work of GAMBLES (1949) and KOMAROV and HAIG (1952). On the other hand, MCKERCHER, MCGOWAN, and SAITO (1954) and MCKERCHER, MCGOWAN, and MCCRORY (1957) successfully employed the cross-protection test to establish the common immunological identity of various American strains of bluetongue virus.

Earlier reports suggested the existence of variant strains of virus solely on the basis of clinical evidence of recurrent attacks of the disease or double bands of petechial haemorrhages encountered on the claws of recovered sheep (ALEXANDER cited by GAMBLES, 1949; LIVINGSTON and HARDY, 1964; PRICE, 1954).

With the introduction of an *in vitro* serum-virus neutralization test in tissue culture, the earlier difficulty of establishing the immunological identity of a particular strain of virus has largely been overcome. In a series of neutralization tests conducted in roller tube cultures of primary lamb kidney cells, 23 strains of virus including the majority of those used by NEITZ (1948), were classified into 12 distinct immunological groups (HOWELL, 1960).

In these tests sheep convalescent sera were used and some slight cross-neutralization between heterologous strains of virus was apparent, but in subsequent plaque inhibition tests with type-specific hyperimmune guinea pig sera, these cross-reactions were virtually eliminated. These results were confirmed by cross-neutralization tests in suckling mice, using mouse-adapted strains and convalescent sheep sera.

In recent years, the examination of numerous field strains from seasonal epizootics, has revealed the existence of an additional 4 immunological groups. The validity of the grouping has been confirmed repeatedly by the classification of a large number of virulent field strains into one or other of the established groups. An index of the selected prototype strains, their identification and origin is given in Table 2.

Table 2. Identification and Origin of Prototype Strains of Bluetongue Virus

| Immuno-logical group No. | Strain identification | | Original donor | Locality of epizootic |
	Sample	Year of collection		
1	Biggarsberg	1958	Sheep	Vryheid-Natal
2	22/59	1959	Sheep	Ermelo-Transvaal
3	Sample B	1943	Sheep	Larnaca-Cyprus
4	Vaccine Batch 603	1900	Sheep	— Cape Province
5	Mossop	1953	Sheep	Machadadorp-Transvaal
6	Strathene	1958	Sheep	Vryheid-Natal
7	Utrecht	1955	Sheep	Utrecht-Natal
8	89/59	1959	Sheep	Ermelo-Transvaal
9	University Farm	1942	Sheep	Pretoria-Transvaal
10	91/59	1959	Sheep	Ermelo-Transvaal
11	Nelspoort	1944	Sheep	Nelspoort-Cape Province
12	Byenespoort	1941	Cow	Pretoria-Transvaal
13	160/59	1959	Sheep	Mt. Currie-Natal
14	87/59	1959	Sheep	Ermelo-Transvaal
15	133/60	1960	Heifer	Onderstepoort-Transvaal
16	Pakistan	1960	Sheep	Hazara-West Pakistan

In 1964, LIVINGSTON and HARDY reported the identification of yet another antigenic variant of bluetongue virus. From the results of tests conducted in tissue culture, it was apparent that antisera to strain 100, which has been identified as a type 10, failed to neutralize the variant Station strain. The relationship of this strain to the established immunological groups has not yet been determined.

The origin of the multiplicity of antigenic types remains obscure. HAIG (1959) has postulated a process of antigenic drift which would enable the virus to maintain itself in the presence of a predominantly immune population. On the contrary, available evidence indicates that at least some of the antigenic types are immunologically stable. No apparent antigenic differences have been detected between the strain originally identified by THEILER in the early part of this century, other type 4 virus strains identified in South Africa during the past 12 years or from strains recovered in Israel, from cattle. Antigenic variation within a type may not be apparent from material collected during this relatively short period of time but extensive immunization with this particular strain during the past 50 years might be expected to have hastened this process. Cross-neutralization tests between a group of plaque purified type 1 strains of virus and their homologous guinea pig antisera have failed to show any evidence of antigenic variation by the more sensitive plaque inhibition test, conducted in this laboratory according to the technique described by PLOTKIN, COHEN, and KOPROWSKI (1961) for polio virus subtypes.

C. Distribution of Antigenic Types

The regional and international distribution of the various antigenic types of virus is of importance when considering the epizootiology and the successful prophylactic immunization of susceptible stock against the disease.

Due to the fact that infectivity is retained for years in blood stored in an oxylate-carbolic-glycerine mixture at $4°C$, it has been possible in recent years to identify, by in vitro techniques, many of the strains described by earlier workers and to compare them with strains active in the field at the present time.

In 1943—44 a particularly virulent strain of virus was recovered from an outbreak of bluetongue amongst sheep in Cyprus (Gambles, 1949). This strain which has subsequently been selected as the prototype representing the 3rd antigenic group, has been found to be immunologically identical to numerous isolates recovered between 1939 and 1967 from outbreaks of bluetongue in South Africa. Neutralization tests have confirmed the conclusion made by ALEXANDER (cited by GAMBLES, 1949), that the Mimosa Park strain used in cross-immunity tests at that time was homologous to this virus.

Between 1943 and 1965, Israel has experienced periodic outbreaks of bluetongue amongst sheep and cattle (KOMAROV and GOLDSMIT, 1951; DAFNI, 1966). Virus strains recovered from two of these outbreaks described by KOMAROV and HAIG (1952) and GOLDSMIT and BARZILAI (1965) has subsequently been identified as type 4. To date many strains of similar antigenic character have been recovered from sheep in South Africa.

Strains of virus recovered from naturally infected sheep in California by McKERCHER, McGOWAN, and SAITO (1953), as well as the strains BT8 and BT11 incorporated in a commercially available vaccine in the United States of America were found to be homologous and antigenically indistinguishable from the type 10 strains isolated in South Africa and 3 strains of virus subsequently obtained from cattle and sheep in Portugal in 1956 (MANSO-RIBEIRO and NORONHA, 1958).

Recent epizootics described by GOUMA and STEVENS (1964) and ZAKI (1965) in the U.A.R. have been shown to be caused by strains of virus representing types 1, 4 and 12 (Bluetongue World Reference Centre, 1967).

In the enzootic regions of Africa, particularly in the south where more material has been studied, all but one of the 16 antigenic types have been identified. The only exception to date is the type 16 strain which has only been found in West Pakistan. From the results of the typing of strains of virus recovered from cattle, sheep and wild caught Culicoides, it is apparent that there is an indiscriminate distribution of the various antigenic types in the host and vector population and within an infected area numerous antigenic types may appear simultaneously in outbreaks of disease amongst susceptible animals (OWEN, DU TOIT, and HOWELL, 1965; HOWELL, 1966). Notwithstanding the apparent random distribution of the various strains amongst the vector population, only a single strain of virus and its subsequent homologous antibody, has been found in the circulation of an individual animal at a particular time following natural infection (HOWELL, KÜMM, and BOTHA, in press). On the other hand, it has been possible to demonstrate the simultaneous circulation of more than one strain of virus in an animal experimentally infected by the intravenous inoculation of polyvalent vaccine.

VI. Interactions with Mammalian Hosts

A. Pathogenesis

After the introduction of the virus into the peripheral circulation it is believed that localised multiplication takes place during the incubation period. This is followed by a viraemia and further distribution of the virus to other sites of predilection where further cycles of multiplication take place. While confirmatory experimental evidence is lacking, the general principles of pathogenesis established for the arthropod borne viruses must be considered applicable to this disease. The first clinically detectable symptom is a rise in temperature when virus is present in the peripheral circulation in highest concentration during the ensuing 48 hours. The virus titre of the blood at this time is seldom more than 100 $TCID_{50}$ per 0.1 ml in primary cultures of lamb kidney cells or 25 to 300 PFU per ml by plaque assay using strain L NCTC929 mouse fibroblasts (HOWELL, KÜMM, and BOTHA, in press). Although many factors will determine the infectivity of the blood when measured in any particular system, differences amongst strains appear to be significant. It has been claimed that a single drop of infective blood is sufficient to establish infection in susceptible sheep by the intravenous route (HUTCHEON, 1902). The infective dose required by the insect vector has not been established.

PINI, COACKLEY and OHDER (1966b) showed that most of the virus in the blood of reacting sheep was associated with the buffy coat. Spleen and mesenteric lymph glands appeared to be the most suitable organs for the *post mortem* isolation of virus.

Evidence regarding the persistence of the virus in the peripheral circulation of convalescent sheep and cattle is conflicting. HUTCHEON (1902) reported that blood taken from sheep 50 days after recovery was infective. DU TOIT (1929b) claimed that the virus of bluetongue was present in the blood of recovered sheep for a period of 4 months or possibly longer. At intervals during this period the presence of the virus could not be demonstrated. HAIG (1959) recorded the recovery of virus for a period of at least 20 days in cattle and indicated that both high titre antibody and virus could be demonstrated simultaneously in the serum. This was confirmed by BOWNE, LUEDKE, FOSTER, and JOCHIM (1966) who detected circulating virus in experimentally infected cattle for periods of up to 28 days, while amongst a group of experimentally infected sheep housed in insect proof stables under conditions precluding natural infection, five were found to circulate virus for a period of 35 days and two exhibited a viraemia for 49 days.

On the other hand ALEXANDER, NEITZ, ADELAAR, and HAIG (1947) and ALEXANDER (1959), maintained that the viraemia in sheep usually does not last for more than a few days after the peak of the febrile reaction, although occasionally circulating virus may be demonstrable for periods not exceeding a few weeks. This contention led to the belief that recovered sheep did not constitute an important reservoir of infection. While the earlier reported observations were subject to the criticism that natural reinfection by heterologous strains could not be excluded, the more recent experimental findings cannot be invalidated on this account. From the results published by Owen, du Toit, and Howell (1966) similar conclusions regarding the persistence of the virus in cattle might well have been made, if not for the fact that further detailed examination of the virus samples showed that the prolonged periods of viraemia were due to repeated reinfection by heterologous strains, followed in each case by a specific immunological response. An irrefutable assessment of this important epizootiological feature of the disease requires the development of a more sensitive assay system.

A study of the excretion of virus by infected animals similarly requires a suitably sensitive assay system. Possibly this aspect has not received much attention since it is generally accepted that biological or mechanical transmission by haematophagous insects is the exclusive method of virus transfer under conditions of field exposure. The single report of Jochim, Luedke, and Bowne (1965) that sheep may become infected following subcutaneous inoculation of urine from sheep experimentally infected with bluetongue virus, indicates that the virus may be shed and remain infective in excretions under suitable conditions.

The pathological lesions indicate that the virus has a predilection for the epithelium of the buccal, nasal and intestinal mucosa as well as the striated musculature.

On the basis of their work on the levels of plasma enzymes in sheep infected with bluetongue virus, Clark and Wagner (1967) suggested that skeletal muscle, myocard and liver were the main organs involved. The fact that creatinine phosphokinase reached very high levels in many cases indicated that skeletal myopathy was an important syndrome of the disease. The absence of significant electrocardiographic abnormalities excluded the myocard as a major source of the increased enzyme levels. The absence of hyperbilirubinaemia and a rise in arginase together with a normal bromsulphthalein excretion excluded acute liver pathology in the pathogenesis of the disease (Clark, 1966).

Schultz and De Lay (1955) incriminated the egg attenuated vaccine virus (Type 10) as the cause of death of lambs born of ewes vaccinated during the 4th to 8th week of pregnancy. It was suggested that the virus invaded the foetal brain and was responsible for cerebral hypoplasia, haemorrhages as well as inflammatory and degenerative changes. Some lambs showed a hydropericard and haemorrhages on the heart and thymus. Griner and McCrory (1964) have also incriminated bluetongue virus infection with abnormalities in newborn lambs.

Similar lesions have been produced experimentally (Young and Cordy, 1964). Lesions in the foetal brain varied from hydroencephaly and subcortical cerebral cysts to a non-suppurative meningo-encephalitis. Richards and Cordy (1967) have suggested that the nervous system of immunologically immature foetal lambs respond to infection by developing congenital abnormalities or necrotising lesions, whereas the brains of older foetuses with greater immunological maturity respond with an inflammatory lesion.

B. Essential Clinical Features

The clinical symptoms of bluetongue in the highly susceptible breeds of sheep have been described in detail by the earlier workers (Spreull, 1905; Theiler, 1906 and Curasson, 1952).

The incubation period following natural infection by the insect vector has not been determined. A single experimental case reported by du Toit (1944) reacted 7 days after allowing wild caught *Culicoides* to feed on the animal. The seasonal termination of the disease with the onset of severe frosts and the resulting reduction of the insect population, suggests that where biological transmission is concerned, the incubation period does not exceed 6 to 7 days. The incubation period following the experimental injection of infective material is subject to many variables. Thus earlier workers, who selected an arbitrary volume of 1 to 2 ml of blood as the means of establishing infection, recorded incubation periods of between 5 to 8 days, although in more exceptional cases this was as short as 2 days or as long as 15 days. Strains of virus attenuated by serial passage in fertile eggs and administered subcutaneously at a dosage level of 10^{-4} TCID$_{50}$ have given a fairly consistent incubation period of 10 days.

The first symptom that is noticed is a sudden or gradual elevation in temperature extending over a period of 48 hours and eventually reaching a peak of 40 to 41°C. The febrile reaction is variable and after reaching an initial peak it fluctuates between 39 and 40°C over a period of 6 to 8 days. The termination of the febrile reaction is determined by the course of the disease and the extent of secondary infection. In animals which recover it seldom exceeds 12 days. Of significance to the clinician is the fact that the character of the febrile reaction has little if any relationship to the severity of the clinical symptoms which are exhibited during the early stages of the disease. An almost imperceptible fever of 39.5°C may be accompanied by the most severe symptoms and death, while a sudden rise to 41°C may be followed by only mild symptoms and recovery.

Within 24 to 36 hours after the first rise in temperature a distinct hyperaemia of the buccal and nasal mucosa develops. This may also be observed in the skin over the ears or where the wool is very short. Shortly afterwards licking movements of the tongue and a mild salivation and frothing may be seen at the corners of the mouth accompanied by a watery discharge from the nostrils and less frequently from the eyes. Over the next few days this discharge becomes more prolific, muco-catarrhal and occasionally mixed with blood.

After about 48 hours the lips and tongue become swollen. This oedema also involves the face to a variable extent and may occasionally include the ears, the lower mandible and extend for a short distance down the ventral surface of the neck. The visible areas of hyperaemia deepen in colour and the papillae in the mouth become acutely reddened. At the same time small petechial haemorrhages appear on the mucous membrane of the mouth, muzzle and in the conjunctiva. In a small percentage of cases this discolouration deepens to an almost purplish blue and the appearance of the tongue gives rise to the popular description of the disease.

Some 5 to 8 days after the first rise in temperature, areas of the mucous membrane of the gums, cheeks and tongue become necrotic leaving exposed, irregularly outlined ulcers, 2 to 4 cm in size and with a haemorrhagic base. They are found opposite the molar teeth and other sites where pressure or friction occurs. In severe cases the tongue becomes gangrenous and an extensive loss of epithelium is experienced. Healing is slow and takes place under a diphtheritic membrane. As a result of these lesions, the saliva becomes mixed with blood and a most offensive odour is given off from the mouth. By this stage the mucopurulent nasal discharge dries in crusts around the nostrils and interferes with breathing. The animal stops feeding as a result of pain arising from the excoriations in the mouth and the swollen tongue; it becomes depressed and assumes a recumbent position with the head doubled around to one side. Ruminal atony develops and the faeces are covered with mucous. In many fatal cases a profuse haemorrhagic diarrhoea is seen.

Towards the end of the febrile reaction, examination of the claws reveal a reddening of the coronary bands, which is more pronounced on the bulbs and more frequently present in the hind feet especially in sheep with unpigmented claws. The feet are warm and painful when pressure is applied. These lesions are more severe in animals on natural grazing than in sheep stabled for experimental purposes. As the inflammatory process continues, the discolouration of the coronary bands becomes darker and a variable number of pinpoint dark red foci appear on the periople. These haemorrhages later become streaky as blood effuses into the horny tubules. These lesions are always bilaterally distributed. As a result of the pain the affected animal stands with an arched back and shows a disinclination to move. In walking it exhibits a stiff gait with varying degrees of lameness and may even be observed to walk on its knees.

There is rapid emaciation due to inanition and the specific muscular lesions. Animals may linger in this state for up to 10 days before dying of exhaustion.

Sequelae to the disease do not usually follow until some time after the acute stage of the disease has subsided. In most animals the wool fibres break and the fleece is shed from various parts of the body about 3 to 4 weeks after the subsidence of the temperature, giving the animal an untidy appearance. In some animals a torticollis develops. The bands of discolouration on the claws regress and move with the growth of new horn, eventually disappearing after 10 to 12 weeks. Exungulation is only rarely encountered.

LUEDKE, BOWNE, JOCHIM, and DOYLE (1964) described the haematological and gross pathological changes in a mixed age group of sheep experimentally infected with the California 8 (Type 10) strain of bluetongue virus. The incubation period varied from 1 to 7 days and the first consistent sign of disease was a marked increase in the rate of respiration which preceded the rise in temperature by 24 hours and persisted for several days. Vomiting was described as a pronounced symptom and a resulting aspiration pneumonia was considered to be the immediate cause of death in a high percentage of cases.

The signs of disease in other species of ruminants are of a much milder nature and a transient fever which hyperaemia is all that may be discerned. In the enzootic regions, cattle only rarely show clinical evidence of disease and a viraemia is usually the only detectable evidence of infection. On the other hand in areas where the disease has made its first appearance amongst a highly susceptible population, symptoms considered to be typical of the more acute form of the disease have been recorded in cattle (SILVA, 1956; CAMPANO LOPEZ and SANCHEZ BOTIJA, 1958).

C. Pathology
1. Macroscopic Pathology

The gross macroscopic lesions observed during the various stages of the disease and after death have been well-documented by SPREULL (1905); THEILER (1906); THOMAS and NEITZ (1947) and MOULTON (1961). The classical description of the disease is associated with the acute febrile and immediate post febrile phase and should be distinguished from the debility and secondary complications such as bronchopneumonia and ruminal atony which follow some time later and are associated more frequently with a fatal outcome. There is no experimental evidence available to indicate either the primary or secondary sites of virus multiplication and the subsequent distribution of the virus in the various tissues of the body. The primary changes are those indicative of an inflammatory process, with an increased permeability of the vascular bed. Evidence of this inflammatory reaction may be found in the digestive, respiratory and locomotory systems. As suggested by MOULTON (1961) the distribution of lesions in sheep with blue-tongue indicates that a wide range of tissues are suitable for virus multiplication.

In the digestive tract the most prominent lesions are those affecting the mouth, where the mucous membrane is oedematous, hyperaemic and later cyanotic. Excoriations develop on the lips, dental pad, the sides and ventral surface of the tongue and on the internal surface of the cheeks opposite the molar teeth. Secondary bacterial invasion is responsible for the diphtheritic necrosis which characterises these ulcers. The forestomachs and oesophageal groove show hyperaemia which is most pronounced on the papillae and laminae. The mucous membrane of the abomasum is oedematous and diffusely hyperaemic, particularly in the proximity of the pylorus. In the small intestine the inflammatory changes vary from mild localised areas of hyperaemia to an extensive catarrhal or haemorrhagic process extending into the large intestine.

The nasal mucous membrane is at first congested and then develops a catarrhal inflammation. Petechial haemorrhages and erosions are frequently found on the skin of the muzzle. The pharyngeal mucous membrane is oedematous and the presence of froth in the trachea will depend upon the extent to which oedema and congestion have developed in the lungs. The frequency of this pathological process and any associated hydrothorax appears to differ amongst the clinical cases described by different authors. Amongst the particular group of sheep studied by LUEDKE, BOWNE, JOCHIM, and DOYLE (1964), aspiration pneumonia, characterised by a reddish purple discoloration and oedema of the lungs, appears to have been a particularly prominent lesion.

Wasting of the musculature constitutes the most important pathological change. The intermuscular fasciae is infiltrated with a clear reddish fluid, giving a gelatinous moist appearance. Haemorrhages of 1 to 2 mm in extent are scattered at random in one or more muscles. These lesions are irregularly distributed and may on occasions measure up to 0.5 cm in size. Pronounced degenerative changes are characterised by the presence of a diffuse opacity or cloudiness, which in some cases may be so severe as to give a grey mottled appearance to the muscle.

In mild cases the pedal lesions in unpigmented claws can be identified as no more than a mild hyperaemia. More frequently this reddening is accompanied by numerous small pin-point foci of haemorrhages on the coronet, which later coalesce to form red vertical streaks within the horny substance. These lesions, if present, are more pronounced in the hind feet and develop earlier than in the fore feet. If the claw is split a marked congestion can be clearly seen in the sensitive laminae.

The extent to which the skin is involved will depend upon the length of the fleece, the presence of pigment and the intensity of any exposure to sunlight. Amongst sheep on range there is generalised reddening of the skin. Where exposure is more severe, irregular exanthematous lesions or even excoriations may develop on the legs and other parts of the body subject to abrasions.

In the cardio-vascular system, the heart is invariably affected to some degree. Petechiae, ecchymoses and necrosis may be present in the myocard and petechial haemorrhages are frequently seen on the endo- and epicardium. A pathonomonic subintimal haemorrhage is observed at the base of the pulmonary artery in most affected animals. A slight hydrothorax, hydropericard and ascites may be seen, but is not a particularly constant feature.

American workers consider necrosis of the papillary muscle of the left ventricle as one of the lesions of major diagnostic importance. As this area of involvement is located deep within the muscle, it is necessary to incise directly across it (KENNEDY, 1968).

The spleen shows a slight tumor splenis and the lymph glands are oedematous and swollen. The glands most frequently involved are the pharyngeal, cervical and thoracic. The liver shows no consistent involvement apart from a mild venous congestion and slight degenerative changes. Similarly, the kidneys are only mildly hyperaemic and oedematous.

NEITZ and RIEMERSCHMID (1944) demonstrated the detrimental influence of solar radiation on the clinical course of bluetongue. Groups of sheep exposed to solar radiation, particularly if shorn, showed more intense symptoms and a higher mortality rate than comparative groups housed in stables.

2. Histopathology

From histopathological studies the earliest symptoms appear to be associated with lesions in the epithelium of the upper portion of the respiratory and digestive tracts. A detailed description of the sequence of the changes which takes place in these tissues has been given by BEKKER, DE KOCK, and QUINLAN (1934) and MOULTON (1961). The ulcers and areas of necrosis in the mouth, nares, rumen and oesophageal groove appear to be the result of a swelling and ballooning of the cells of the striated epithelium. In these cells accumulations of large acidophilic intracytoplasmic masses can be demonstrated and are followed by pyknosis and disintegration of the nucleus. The cell destruction is followed by the infiltration of neutrophiles into these artificially created spaces. The ulceration and necrosis extends downwards from the surface to involve all the layers of the stratified epithelium, with the base of the ulcer eventually being formed by the necrotic surface of the corium. During the early stages of the disease the inflammatory response is essentially mild as reflected by the degree of oedema, hyperaemia, haemorrhage and round cell infiltration. In some cases healing is rapid and complete, however, when complicated by secondary bacterial infection, more severe lesions develop and after healing leave well-defined depressions on the surface of the mucous membrane.

THOMAS and NEITZ (1947) described the inflammatory changes observed in the skin and claws. It was reported that the hyperaemia of the vascular corium of the claws was essentially a continuation of the process taking place in the skin. The papillary bodies, especially at their tips, were found to be the seat of intense vascular engorgement, which gave rise to a serous exudation and extravasation. The typical red streaks seen in the horn of the claws in close proximity to the coronet were due to the filling of the hollow medullary canals of the horny wall with extravasated erythrocytes and polymorphonuclear leucocytes.

By far the most important although inconsistent pathological changes are those involving the striated musculature. THOMAS and NEITZ (1947) recognised five distinct stages in the development of the muscular lesions, characterised by differential staining, swelling and distortion, breaking up and resorption, intramuscular haemorrhages and finally regeneration of the muscle fibres. It was emphasised that all or some of these changes could be found at the same time in the same muscle.

The earliest evidence of degeneration is a change in the staining reaction of formalin-fixed sections stained with haemalum-eosin. The affected fibres appear deep reddish purple in colour in contrast to the pale mauve of normal fibres. In the affected muscles a coagulation of the sarcoplasm produces irregular swollen and bulging fibres. This distortion distinguishes them from the otherwise normal regular wavy fibres. Shrinkage of the sarcoplasm leaves a length of emptied sarcolemma. As a result of hyalinisation the cross striations disappear early, although they may persist until the sarcoplasm disintegrates and becomes phagocytosed. Pyknosis of the sarcolemma may be seen, but rarely proceeds to complete necrosis. With the breaking up of the fibres, numerous histiocytes or macrophages invade the affected areas and liquify most of the sarcoplasm. Occasionally portions of such sarcoplasm become calcified. Haemorrhages which occur either in or near foci of degeneration vary in size and are associated with a rupture of the capillaries adjacent to the torn muscle fibres. Regeneration commences with the division of the nuclei of the sarcolemma accompanied by the infiltration of other tissue elements.

From the nature of the proliferative changes THOMAS and NEITZ (1947) believed that the regeneration was genuine. They considered that the pronounced muscular weakness and rapid loss of flesh in affected sheep was essentially due to the disintegration and resorption of the muscle fibres, a process which continued long after the termination of the febrile reaction. Although not clearly defined, they also found that all cases of torticollis were associated with severe localised degeneration of the cervical muscles. It appeared that the damage was more extensive on the side toward which the head was bent. A persistent torticollis following recovery from bluetongue was considered to be due to a fibrous replacement of the damaged muscle.

Essentially similar pathological changes in the myocardium were described by MOULTON (1961). In sheep showing haemorrhage in the pulmonary artery the accumulation of blood was most frequently found in the media and less frequently in the adventitia.

BWANGAMOI (1965) has described the pathology of ovine foetuses infected with bluetongue virus. The primary lesions observed included a generalised oedema and hyperaemia, haemorrhages in the liver, adrenal medulla and heart, focal necrosis of the myocardium and a non-suppurative meningitis of the brain and spinal cord. While encephalopathy similar to that observed with the vaccine virus was also recorded, the effect of the virulent virus differed from that of the attenuated vaccine virus in so far as a generalised necrosis of the liver and suppressed hepatic haematopoiesis was evident, together with specific embryo mortality.

3. Clinical Pathology

A general increase in blood sugar, non-protein nitrogen and urea nitrogen fractions in the blood of sheep suffering from bluetongue was reported by GRAF (1933). In severe clinical cases, a decrease in haemoglobin and a corresponding decrease in total nitrogen was apparent. The extent of variations amongst the values obtained correspond approximately to the severity of the reaction.

In free electrophoretic studies, MANSO-RIBEIRO and NORONHA (1958) demonstrated a marked increase in the gamma globulin fraction of serum from diseased sheep.

In a preliminary communication CLARK (1966) reported that the plasma levels of glutamic oxalacetic transaminase (GOT), glutamic pyruvic transaminase (GPT), lactic dehydrogenase (LDH) and aldolase (ALD) rose after the subsidence of the fever reaction in bluetongue. Peak levels were found some 8 days after the peak of the febrile reactions and elevated levels persisted for some 8 days thereafter.

Subsequently the plasma enzyme levels of six sheep in the acute stages of the disease were studied by CLARK and WAGNER (1967). In those animals which ultimately died from the disease, a significant increase in aldolase, lactic dehydrogenase, creatine phosphokinase, glutamic oxalacetic transaminase and glutamic pyruvic transaminase was demonstrated. Amongst a group of 18 convalescent animals the most consistent increases in enzyme levels were found to involve glutamic pyruvic transaminase and aldolase. In experimentally infected sheep, LUEDKE, BOWNE, JOCHIM, and DOYLE (1964) found that a leucopenia was detectable 48 hours before the maximum rise in body temperature. Neutropenia, lymphopenia and eosinopenia were present in a high percentage of affected animals. The decreased lymphocyte and leucocyte curves closely paralleled one another, whereas neutrophile and eosinophile depressions occurred primarily during the convalescent stages of the disease. Haemolytic anaemia occurred in all but one of the experimental animals.

D. Immunity

1. Immunological Response to Bluetongue Virus

The administration of a given volume of preserved infective blood has been the method most frequently used to challenge the immunity of recovered experimental animals. Following challenge, an arbitrary system of scoring was used to indicate the character of the febrile reaction and the extent to which pathological lesions developed. This empirical procedure, using either homologous or heterologous strains of virus, was exclusively employed by the earlier workers including THEILER (1906); DU TOIT (1929a); NEITZ (1948) and McKERCHER, McGOWAN, and McCRORY (1957). In more recent unpublished experiments in this laboratory, an alternate and more sensitive method of challenge has been used. This technique involved the intravenous administration of 10,000 $TCID_{50}$ of tissue culture adapted virus, followed by daily sampling of blood to establish the presence of viraemia, by either qualitative or quantitative assay in a suitable tissue culture system. Although clinical evidence of disease was invariably restricted to a febrile reaction of short duration, a good relationship was obtained between circulating virus and the presence or absence of neutralizing antibody at the time of challenge.

The rise and persistence of antibodies or immunity to bluetongue virus has been the subject of investigation by various techniques. DU TOIT (1929a) conclude from challenge experiments that there was a gradual, yet slow decrease in immunity from 3rd to 12th month following recovery from infection. NEITZ (1948) was unable to confirm this observation and suggested that challenge of the immune sheep by a heterologous strain could have accounted for the apparent short duration of immunity.

Biochemical characterization of the bluetongue antibody has not been reported. While neutralizing and precipitating antibody is stable at 56° C, inactivation of sera for complement fixation tests at this temperature has revealed a rapid loss of activity and may account for the low titres reported by some workers.

Neutralizing antibody has been detected as early as 4 to 8 days after experimental infection with virulent virus (KLONTZ, SVEHAG, and GORHAM, 1962). JOCHIM, LUEDKE, and BOWNE (1965) reported the presence of antibodies on the 14th day after infection. Peak antibody titres appear to develop by the 30th day and persist for a period of at least 12 months but are probably lifelong.

Complement fixing antibodies may be detected as early as the 10th day after the first rise in temperature, increasing to a peak level by the 36th day and persisting for 6 to 8 weeks, after which they disappear rapidly from the circulation and are no longer present in significant titre after 12 months. In view of the group-specific reactivity of the antigen and the persistence of the precipitating antibody it appears that the agar gel diffusion test is a more reliable technique for the screening of experimental animals for susceptibility to bluetongue (KLONTZ, SVEHAG, and GORHAM, 1962).

The reports of the isolation of virus and the identification of homologous neutralizing antibody simultaneously from the blood of cattle are of particular interest with regard to the epizootiology of the disease (HAIG, 1959; BOWNE, LUEDKE, FOSTER, and JOCHIM, 1966). The presence of circulating antibody does not appear to prevent reinfection by heterologous strains. NEITZ (1948) concluded that the immunity against one strain of virus does not interfere with the antigenic stimulus provided by another strain.

In practice a great deal of variation has been encountered in the titres of both neutralizing and complement-fixing antibodies between individual animals. The frequent occurrence of anticomplementary activity in sheep sera and the identification of non-specific inhibitors in some calf sera has been reported (PINI, COACKLEY, and OHDER, 1966a).

After the administration of egg attenuated strains of virus, neutralizing antibodies are present in low titre, but would appear to be effective in preventing natural infection from the 10th day after immunization. Low titre complement fixing antibodies could be detected in sheep following the administration of an egg attenuated strain of virus (MCKERCHER, MCGOWAN, and SAITO, 1954).

Newborn lambs acquire a passive immunity from immune ewes through the ingestion of colostrum within 24 hours after birth. NEITZ (1948) showed that it persisted for a period of between 4 and 68 days. HAIG (1959) claimed that lambs from susceptible dams have some natural resistance, whereas lambs from immune dams have a high degree of immunity that may persist for 68 days or more. Unpublished work by WEISS (V. R. I. Onderstepoort, personal communication) has shown that colostral immunity persists for a period of up to 6 months after birth and interferes with the immunological response following the administration of live attenuated vaccines. LIVINGSTON and HARDY (1957) found that this interference persisted for a period of up to 2 weeks after weaning. SVEHAG and GORHAM (1963) studied the passive transfer of immunity to bluetongue virus from vaccinated female mice to their offspring. They considered that only lacteal transfer of neutralizing antibody took place from the immune mothers to their offspring, although the *in utero* transfer of antibody at a very low level, could not be excluded. After weaning, the passive immunity was lost at a rate consistent with the reported half-life for mouse antibody. These authors suggested that the immunological relationships between strains of bluetongue virus, might possibly be assessed, by using a cross protection type of test in infant mice, born of vaccinated mothers.

2. Active Immunization

The attempts of earlier workers at prophylactic immunization are of no more than historical interest and have little bearing on current vaccines in use. Various aspects of these earlier vaccines and their use in the field have been reviewed elsewhere (ALEXANDER, NEITZ, ADELAAR, and HAIG, 1947; NEITZ, 1948; COX, 1954; HAIG, 1959). Modifications in the techniques of production have been described in greater detail by KEMENY and DREHLE (1961) and HOWELL (1963).

Effective prophylactic immunization constitutes one of the most challenging problems in current research. Under certain circumstances, where it has been established that only a single or otherwise a limited number of strains of virus are active in a region, a monovalent live attenuated vaccine developed from the local strain has proved very successful. MCKERCHER, MCGOWAN, CABASSO, ROBERTS, and SAITO (1957) have described the development, safety testing, potency and stability of a modified live virus vaccine employing American strains of bluetongue virus. In an extensive field trial with the attenuated California strain on 10,000 sheep, 92% of 3% of the sheep which were challenged 6 weeks following vaccination, showed complete protection and only 0.4% exhibited a severe reaction (MCGOWAN and MCKERCHER, 1954).

On the other hand a polyvalent vaccine prepared from four strains of egg attenuated virus proved highly successful in controlling the spread of bluetongue through the Iberian Peninsula, where a fifth heterologous strain was involved (CAMPANO LOPEZ and SANCHEZ BOTIJA, 1958; MANSO-RIBEIRO and NORONHA, 1958).

In the enzootic regions of Africa, where numerous antigenic types of virus may be active during an epizootic in any particular area, control is more difficult. As a result, a polyvalent live attenuated vaccine has to be employed, with the associated problems resulting from the interference between strains, differences in immunizing potency, growth rates of the modified strains and the marked differences in the response of individual animals to such vaccines.

E. Epizootiology

Although confused over the etiology of the disease, HUTCHEON (1902) recognised similarities in the environmental conditions under which both horsesickness and bluetongue occurred. It was recognised at that time that climatic and farming practices had an important influence on the incidence of the disease. In very dry seasons bluetongue was less prevalent, whereas in seasons when there was an abundance of rain the disease would appear over a very large area of the country, irrespective of the altitude above sea level. Sheep were considered to be protected against the disease if they were housed at night and were not allowed to graze until well after sunrise. He also obtained convincing evidence of the role of an insect vector in the transmission of bluetongue, by observing the reduced incidence of the disease after the dipping of sheep in an insecticide.

SPREULL (1905) also noted the distinct seasonal incidence of the disease and observed that bluetongue was more common in paddocks situated in valleys or near rivers, dams and marshy places thus emphasizing the importance of humidity. A significant observation was the fact that outbreaks ceased to occur after the first frosts. This author produced further circumstantial evidence to support the role of an insect vector and concluded that the epizootiology was intimately bound up with the life history of some insect. THEILER (1906), after summarising these facts, appeared convinced of the role of an insect vector, but also expressed interest in the survival of the virus during interepizootic periods. All of the earlier workers were emphatic that the disease was not contagious.

The first transmission experiments with bluetongue virus were reported in 1934 (NIESCHULZ, BEDFORD, and DU TOIT). From preliminary studies and a consideration of epizootiological facts, these authors believed that Aedes species of mosquitoes might be responsible. Although virus was apparently recovered on 3 occasions from mosquitoes previously fed on infected sheep, the evidence was not convincing and no biological cycle was established.

DU TOIT (1944) described a series of experiments in which pools of wild caught *Culicoides*, when emulsified and injected into susceptible sheep, produced clinical evidence of bluetongue. In another experiment, the disease was produced by the bites of wild caught *Culicoides*, which had been allowed to feed 10 days previously on a sheep reacting to bluetongue. The species considered responsible for this transmission was identified as *C. pallidipennis* (Carter, Ingram and Macfie). PRICE and HARDY (1954) similarly reported the successful transmissio of bluetongue to sheep on two separate occasions by injecting emulsions of wild caught culicoides, of the species *C. variipennis* (Coquillett).

The most convincing evidence of the role of culicoides species in the transmission of bluetongue to date, is that which has been presented by FOSTER, JONES, and McCRORY (1963). With colonised *C. variipennis*, 5 positive biological transmissions were reported under controlled laboratory conditions. Insects were maintained for periods of 10 to 15 days after ingestion of the virus before being allowed to refeed on susceptible sheep. Transmission was not obtained with insects in which the intrinsic incubation period was less than 10 days. These authors reported that both transmission and isolation trials with *Aedes aegypti* (Linneaus) and *Stomoxys calcitrans* (Linneaus) were negative.

By electron microscopy BOWNE and JONES (1966) have demonstrated the replicative cycle of bluetongue virus in the salivary glands of *C. variipennis*. JOCHIM and JONES (1966) have produced evidence to show that the virus will multiply in *C. variipennis* after intrathoracic inoculation. The most rapid increase in virus concentration occurred within the first 48 hours, with an approximate twentyfold increase in titre. After 5 to 8 days incubation the average increase was of the order of ten-thousandfold. The transmission of the virus by inoculated *C. variipennis* to embryonated chicken eggs has been described by JONES and FOSTER (1966).

GRAY and BANNISTER (1961) showed that the sheep ked *Melophagus ovinus* (Linneaus) collected from reacting sheep could harbour the virus. Further investigations by LUEDKE, JOCHIM, and BOWNE (1965) confirmed that the ked could transmit the disease, but it was not possible to determine whether this was a true biological or purely mechanical transmission. From these findings sufficient evidence has been produced to stimulate further investigation of the possible role of this vector.

While much attention has been given to the role of the insect vector in the transmission of the disease, other methods of virus transfer have been generally discredited. JOCHIM, LUEDKE, and BOWNE (1965) produced evidence to suggest that sheep may become infected by repeated oral administration of bluetongue virus, thus creating the possibility of infection between sheep during continued contact.

Apart from the role of the insect vector in the epizootiology of bluetongue, the interplay of many factors have a bearing on the distribution and incidence of the disease (DU TOIT, 1962; LUEDKE, JONES, and JOCHIM, 1967; HOWELL, 1966).

Bluetongue is essentially a disease of sheep and was only recognised when highly susceptible animals of this species were introduced into enzootic areas. An assessment of the susceptibility of various breeds of sheep, on the basis of the severity of the clinical symptoms, has shown that the European breeds, particularly the Dorset Horn, are highly susceptible compared to the African and Asiatic breeds such as the Black Head Persian and Karakul. The Merino is less susceptible than the Dorset Horn (NEITZ, 1948). A marked variation in the susceptibility of individual animals and the variation in the virulence of naturally occurring strains of virus are responsible for the unpredictable mortality encountered amongst flocks during widespread epizootics.

In addition to sheep, other ruminants are susceptible to bluetongue. SPREULL (1905) showed that calves could be infected artificially, while BEKKER, DE KOCK, and QUINLAN (1934), DE KOCK, DU TOIT and NEITZ (1937), and DU TOIT (1962) reported the recovery of virus from bovines exposed to natural infection. Earlier workers (MASON and NEITZ, 1940) came to the conclusion that infective blood, when administered by various routes, does not cause apparent signs of illness in cattle. During the course of recent epizootics of bluetongue outside Africa classical symptoms of bluetongue have nevertheless been described in cattle (KOMAROV and GOLDSMIT, 1951; SILVA, 1956; CAMPANO LOPEZ and SANCHEZ BOTIJA, 1958). Goats apparently possess the same degree of susceptibility as cattle. Clinical symptoms have been produced experimentally in goats and have also been observed by farmers during natural outbreaks of the disease (SPREULL, 1905; KOMAROV and GOLDSMIT, 1951).

In view of the susceptibility of domesticated ruminants, it is believed that a wide variety of antelope will also experience a viraemia without the manifestation of clinical symptoms. NEITZ (1933) experimentally infected two blesbucks *Damaliscus albifrons* and succeeded in recovering virus between the 8th and 17th days. In both these experimental animals the infection was inapparent. An unpublished report (YOUNG, Vet. Lab. Skukuza, personal communication) described an acute and fatal case of bluetongue in buffalo calves infected experimentally. Bluetongue has also been described in deer (ROBINSON, STAIR, and JONES, 1967; VOSDINGH, TRAINER, and EASTERDAY, 1968), the topi, *Damaliscus karrigum ugandae* (WELLS, 1962) and the desert bighorn sheep (ROBINSON, HAILEY, LIVINGSTON, and THOMAS, 1967).

Solipeds, dogs, cats, ferrets, rabbits and guinea pigs are apparently insusceptible to bluetongue virus.

VII. Classification and Nomenclature

Because of its transmission by an arthropod vector, the virus of bluetongue was first classified in the arbovirus group (CASALS, 1959). For some years, however, it has been apparent that certain characteristics were not typically those of an arbovirus and inclusion in this family has been questioned. The better known arboviruses are all sensitive to ether and deoxycholate, a characteristic usually accepted to indicate the presence of a lipid-containing envelope. Electron microscopy at first did not resolve the question, as both OWEN and MUNZ (1966) and BOWNE and JONES (1966) described the presence of an envelope. Subsequently this envelope was shown to be an artifact (LECATSAS, 1968; ELS and VERWOERD, 1969). STUDDERT, PANGBORN, and ADDISON (1966) suggested a reovirus-like structure for the capsid, with 92 capsomeres in icosahedral arrangement. ANDREWES and PEREIRA (1967) provisionally classified both bluetongue virus and the related African horsesickness virus as reoviruses on the basis of this structure.

Studies of the physico-chemical characteristics of the virus and especially the finding that its genome consists of a double-stranded RNA, almost indistinguishable from reovirus RNA, seemed to confirm this deduction (VERWOERD, 1969). However, high resolution electron micrographs obtained by negative staining of highly purified virus revealed that the bluetongue virion is smaller than reovirus and that its capsid contains 32 (or possibly 42) but definitely not 92 capsomeres. No evidence for a double capsid was found. On morphological grounds, therefore, the bluetongue virus can be considered as distinct from the reoviruses (ELS and VERWOERD, 1969).

Other differences between the two viruses include a lack of serological cross reaction and a pronounced difference in both thermal and pH stability. There would appear to be no doubt that some relationship between the two groups does exist, but that bluetongue virus cannot be regarded as a typical reovirus.

To project these conclusions into the classification system as presently used, VERWOERD (1968) proposed the creation of a new group, termed Diplorna viruses (in analogy to Picorna viruses) to include both reo- and bluetongue viruses as well as several other agents under investigation.

References

ALEXANDER, R. A.: The propagation of bluetongue virus in the developing chick embryo with particular reference to the temperature of incubation. Onderstepoort J. vet. Sci. Anim. Ind. 22, 7—26 (1947).

ALEXANDER, R. A.: Bluetongue as an international problem. Bull. Off. int. Epiz. 51, 432—439 (1959).

ALEXANDER, R. A., and D. A. HAIG: The use of egg attenuated bluetongue virus in the production of a polyvalent vaccine for sheep. A. Propagation of the virus in sheep. Onderstepoort J. vet. Res. 25, 3—15 (1951).

ALEXANDER, R. A., D. A. HAIG, and T. F. ADELAAR: The attenuation of bluetongue virus by serial passage through fertile eggs. Onderstepoort J. vet. Sci. Anim. Ind. 21, 231—241 (1947).

ALEXANDER, R. A., W. O. NEITZ, T. F. ADELAAR, and D. A. HAIG: A review of the bluetongue problem. J. S. Afr. vet. med. Ass. 18, 51—58 (1947).

ANDREWES, C.: Viruses of Vertebrates. First edition. Baillière, Tindall and Cassell, London (1964).

ANDREWES, C., and H. G. PEREIRA: Viruses of Vertebrates. Second edition. Baillière, Tindall and Cassell, London, 1967.

BEKKER, J. G., G. DE KOCK, and J. B. QUINLAN: The occurrence and identification of bluetongue in cattle: the so-called pseudo foot-and-mouth disease in South Africa. Onderstepoort J. vet. Sci. 2, 393—507 (1934).

BELLAMY, A. R., L. SHAPIRO, J. T. AUGUST, and W. K. JOKLIK: Studies on reovirus RNA. I. Characterization of reovirus genome RNA. J. molec. Biol. 29, 1—17 (1967).

Bluetongue World Reference Centre. Report (1967).

BOULANGER, P.: Technique of a modified direct complement-fixation test for viral antibodies in heat inactivated cattle serum. Canad. J. comp. Med. 24, 262—269 (1960).

BOULANGER, P., G. M. RUCKERBAUER, G. L. BANNISTER, D. P. GRAY, and A. GIRARD: Studies on Bluetongue. III. Comparison of two complement-fixation methods. Canad. J. comp. Med. 31, 166—170 (1967).

BOWNE, J. G., and M. M. JOCHIM: Cytopathologic changes and development of inclusion bodies in cultured cells infected with bluetongue virus. Amer. J. vet. Res. 28, 1091—1106 (1967).

BOWNE, J. G., and R. H. JONES: Observations on bluetongue virus in the salivary glands of an insect vector, Culicoides variipennis. Virology 30, 127—133 (1966).

BOWNE, J. G., A. J. LUEDKE, N. M. FOSTER, and M. M. JOCHIM: Current aspects of bluetongue in cattle. J. Amer. vet. med. Ass. 148, 1177—1180 (1966).

BOWNE, J. G., A. J. LUEDKE, M. M. JOCHIM, and N. M. FOSTER: Current status of bluetongue in sheep. J. Amer. vet. med. Ass. 144, 759—764 (1964).

BWANGAMOI, O.: Pathology of ovine foetuses in bluetongue virus infection. Diss. Abstr. 27B, 2001 (1966).

CABASSO, V. J., G. I. ROBERTS, J. M. DOUGLAS, R. ZORZI, M. R. STEBBINS, and H. R. COX: Bluetongue. 1. Propagation of bluetongue virus of sheep in suckling hamsters. Proc. Soc. exp. Biol. (N.Y.) 88, 678—681 (1955).

CAMPANO LOPEZ, A., and C. SANCHEZ BOTIJA: Bluetongue in Spain. Bull. Off. int. Epiz. **50**, 67—93 (1958).

CASALS, J.: Antigenic classification of arthropod-borne viruses. Proc. 6th Int. Congr. trop. Med. and Malar. **5**, 34—37 (1959).

CASPAR, D. L. D., and A. KLUG: Physical principles in the construction of regular viruses. Cold Spr. Harb. Symp. quant. Biol. **27**, 1—24 (1962).

CLARK, R.: Plasma enzymes in bluetongue. J. S. Afr. vet. med. Ass. **37**, 452 (1966).

CLARK, R., and ADRIANA M. WAGNER: Plasma enzymes in bluetongue. J. S. Afr. vet. med. Ass. **38**, 221—223 (1967).

COX, H. R.: Bluetongue. Bact. Rev. **18**, 239—253 (1954).

CURASSON, G.: Introduction de la Bluetongue en Afrique Occidentale Française. Bull. Soc. Path. exot. **18**, 215—218 (1925).

DAFNI, I.: Bluetongue in Israel in the years 1964 and 1965. Bull. Off. int. Epiz. **66**, 319—327 (1966).

DE KOCK, G., R. M. DU TOIT, and W. O. NEITZ: Observations on bluetongue in cattle and sheep. Onderstepoort J. vet. Sci. **8**, 129—180 (1937).

DU TOIT, P. J.: The nature and duration of the immunity against bluetongue in sheep. 15th Ann. Rep. Dir. vet. Services. Union of S. Africa. 69—78 (1929a).

DU TOIT, P. J.: Studies on the virus of bluetongue. 15th Ann. rep. Dir. vet. Services. Union of S. Africa. 79—93 (1929b).

DU TOIT, R. M.: The transmission of Blue-Tongue and Horse-sickness by *Culicoides*. Onderstepoort J. vet. Sci. Anim. Ind. **19**, 7—16 (1944).

DU TOIT, R. M.: The role played by bovines in the transmission of bluetongue in sheep. J. S. Afr. vet. med. Ass. **33**, 483—490 (1962).

ELS, H. J., and D. W. VERWOERD: Morphology of the bluetongue virus. Virology **38**, 213—219 (1969).

FAO/OIE: Animal Health Year Book. Food and Agriculture Organisation of the United Nations, Rome, 1964.

FERNANDES, M. V.: Isolation and propagation of bluetongue virus in tissue culture. Amer. J. vet. Res. **20**, 398—408 (1959a).

FERNANDES, M. V.: Cytopathogenic effects of bluetongue virus on lamb tissues *in vitro*. Tex. Rep. Biol. Med. **17**, 94—105 (1959b).

FOSTER, N. M., R. H. JONES, and B. R. MCCRORY: Preliminary investigations on insect transmission of bluetongue virus in sheep. Amer. J. vet. Res. **24**, 1195—1200 (1963).

GAMBLES, R. M.: Bluetongue of sheep in Cyprus. J. comp. Path. **59**, 176—190 (1949).

GIRARD, A., G. M. RUCKERBAUER, D. P. GRAY, G. L. BANNISTER, and P. BOULANGER: Studies on Bluetongue. IV. Studies of three strains in primary bovine foetal kidney cell cultures. Canad. J. comp. Med. **31**, 171—174 (1967).

GOLDSMIT, LEAH, and E. BARZILAI: Isolation and propagation of a bluetongue virus strain in embryonating chicken eggs by the intravenous route of inoculation — preliminary report. Refuah vet. **22**, 285—279 (1965).

GORHAM, J. R.: A simple technique for the inoculation of the chorio-allantoic membrane of chicken embryos. Amer. J. vet. Res. **18**, 691—692 (1957).

GOUMA, I. S., and A. J. STEVENS: An outbreak of suspected bluetongue in sheep in Egypt. J. Arab. vet. med. Ass. **24**, 21—24 (1964).

GRAF, H.: Comparative studies on "laked" and "unlaked" blood filtrates of sheep in health and during "heartwater" (Rickettsia ruminatum) infection and blue-tongue (catarrhal fever). Onderstepoort J. vet. Sci. **1**, 285—334 (1933).

GRAY, D. P., and G. L. BANNISTER: Studies on bluetongue. I. Infectivity of the virus in the sheep ked *Melophagus ovinus* (L). Ganad. J. comp. Med. **25**, 230—232 (1961).

GRINER, L. A., and B. R. MCCRORY: Bluetongue associated with abnormalities in newborn lambs. J. Amer. vet. med. Ass. **145**, 1013—1019 (1964).

HAIG, D. A.: Bluetongue. Proc. 16th Int. Vet. Congr. Madrid, 215—225 (1959).

HAIG, D. A., D. G. MCKERCHER, and R. A. ALEXANDER: The cytopathogenic action of bluetongue virus on tissue cultures and its application to the detection of antibodies in the serum of sheep. Onderstepoort J. vet. Res. **27**, 171—177 (1956).

HARDY, W. T., and D. A. PRICE: Soremuzzle of sheep. J. Amer. vet. med. Ass. **120**, 23—25 (1952).

HENNING, M. W.: Blue-tongue, Bloutong. Animal diseases in South Africa. 2nd ed., Central News Agency, Ltd., South Africa, 1949.

HOWELL, P. G.: A preliminary antigenic classification of strains of bluetongue virus. Onderstepoort J. vet. Res. **28**, 357—363 (1960).

HOWELL, P. G.: Bluetongue. Emerging Disease of Animals. F.A.O. Agricultural Series No. 61, 109—153 (1963).

HOWELL, P. G.: Some aspects of the epizootiology of bluetongue. Bull. Off. int. Epiz. **66**, 341—352 (1966).

HOWELL, P. G., N. A. KÜMM, and M. J. BOTHA: The application of improved techniques to the identification of strains of bluetongue virus. Onderstepoort J. vet. Res. **37**, (1970). (In press.)

HOWELL, P. G., D. W. VERWOERD, and R. A. OELLERMANN: Plaque formation by bluetongue virus. Onderstepoort J. vet. Res. **34**, 317—332 (1967).

HUTCHEON, D.: Fever or epizootic catarrh. Rep. Coll. Vet. Surg. for 1880, 12 (1881).

HUTCHEON, D.: Malarial Catarrhal fever of sheep. Vet. Rec. **14**, 629—633 (1902).

INABA, Y., S. ISHII, and T. OMORI: Bluetongue-like disease in Japan. Bull. Off. int. Epiz. **66**, 329—340 (1966).

ISHITANI, R.: Lesions and the pathological differential diagnosis of a bluetongue-like disease in cattle. J. Jap. vet. med. Ass. **20**, 219—228 (1967) (J).

JOCHIM, M. M., and R. H. JONES: Multiplication of bluetongue virus in *Culicoides variipennis* following artificial infection. Amer. J. Epidem. **84**, 241—246 (1966).

JOCHIM, M. M., A. J. LUEDKE, and J. G. BOWNE: The clinical and immunogenic response of sheep to oral and intradermal administrations of bluetongue virus. Amer. J. vet. Res. **26**, 1254—1260 (1965).

JONES, R. H., and N. M. FOSTER: The transmission of bluetongue virus to embryonating chicken eggs by *Culicoides variipennis* (Diptera: Ceratopogonidae) infected by intrathoracic inoculation. Mosquito News **26**, 184—185 (1966).

KEMENY, L., and L. E. DREHLE: The use of tissue culture-propagated bluetongue virus for vaccine production. Amer. J. vet. Res. **22**, 921—925 (1961).

KENNEDY, P. C.: Some aspects of bluetongue in the United States. Aust. vet. J. **44**, 191—194 (1968).

KIPPS, A.: Complement fixation with antigens prepared from bluetongue virus-infected mouse brains. J. Hyg. (Lond.) **54**, 79—88 (1956).

KIPPS, A.: A study of the soluble antigen of the bluetongue viruses. University of Cape Town (Thesis) (1958).

KLONTZ, G. W., S.-E. SVEHAG, and J. R. GORHAM: A study by the agar diffusion technique of precipitating antibody directed against blue tongue virus and its relation to homotypic neutralising antibody. Arch. ges. Virusforsch. **12**, 259—268 (1962).

KOMAROV, A., and LEAH GOLDSMIT: A disease similar to bluetongue in cattle and sheep in Israel. Refuah vet. **8**, 96—100 (1951).

KOMAROV, A., and D. A. HAIG: Identification of a strain of bluetongue virus isolated in Israel. J. S. Afr. vet. med. Ass. **23**, 153—156 (1952).

LECATSAS, G.: Electron microscopy study of the formation of bluetongue virus. Onderstepoort J. vet. Res. **35**, 139—149 (1968).

LIVINGSTON, C. W., and W. T. HARDY: Isolation of an antigenic variant of bluetongue virus. Amer. J. vet. Res. **25**, 1598—1600 (1964).

LIVINGSTON, C. W., and R. W. MOORE: Cytochemical changes of bluetongue virus in tissue culture. Amer. J. vet. Res. **23**, 701—710 (1962).

LUEDKE, A. J., J. G. BOWNE, M. M. JOCHIM, and CORA DOYLE: Clinical and pathologic features of bluetongue in sheep. Amer. J. vet. Res. **25**, 963—970 (1964).

LUEDKE, A. J., M. M. JOCHIM, and J. G. BOWNE: Preliminary bluetongue transmission with the sheep ked *Melophagus Ovinus* (L). Canad. J. Comp. Med. **29**, 229—231 (1965).

LUEDKE, A. J., R. H. JONES, and M. M. JOCHIM: Transmission of bluetongue between sheep and cattle by *Culicoides variipennis*. Amer. J. vet. Res. **28**, 457—460 (1967).

MANSO-RIBEIRO, J., and F. M. O. NORONHA: Fièvre catarrhale du mouton au Portugal (blue tongue). Bull. Off. int. Epiz. **50,** 46—64 (1958).

MANSO-RIBEIRO, J., J. A. ROSA-AZEVEDO, F. M. O. NORONHA, M. C. BRACOFORTE, JR., C. GRAVE-PEREIRA, and M. VASCO-FERNANDES: Bluetongue in Portugal. Bull. Off. int. Epiz. **48,** 350—367 (1957).

MASON, J. H., J. D. W. A. COLES, and R. A. ALEXANDER: Cultivation of bluetongue virus in fertile eggs produced on a vitamin deficient diet. Nature (Lond.) **145,** 1022—1023 (1940).

MASON, J. H., and W. O. NEITZ: The susceptibility of cattle to the virus of bluetongue. Onderstepoort J. vet. Sci. **15,** 149—157 (1940).

MAYOR, H. D.: Studies on reovirus. III. A labile, single stranded ribonucleic acid associated with the late stages of infection. J. nat. Cancer Inst. **35,** 919—925 (1965).

McCRORY, B. R., N. M. FOSTER, and R. C. BAY: Virucidal effect of some chemical agents on bluetongue virus. Amer. J. vet. Res. **20,** 665—669 (1959).

McGOWAN, B.: An epidemic resembling sore muzzle or bluetongue in California sheep. Cornell Vet. **43,** 213—216 (1953).

McGOWAN, B., and D. G. McKERCHER: Studies on Bluetongue. II. Field experiences with bluetongue in California. Proc. Book Amer. vet. med. Ass. **91,** 61—64 (1954).

McKERCHER, D. G., B. McGOWAN, V. J. CABASSO, G. I. ROBERTS, and J. K. SAITO: Studies on Bluetongue. III. The development of a modified live virus vaccine employing American strains of bluetongue virus. Amer. J. vet. Res. **18,** 310—316 (1957).

McKERCHER, D. G., B. McGOWAN, and B. R. McCRORY: Studies on bluetongue. V. Distribution of bluetongue in the United States as confirmed by diagnostic tests. J. Amer. vet. med. Ass. **130,** 86—89 (1957).

McKERCHER, D. G., B. McGOWAN, and J. K. SAITO: Studies on Bluetongue. I. Isolation, identification, and typing of the bluetongue virus and a preliminary report on the serodiagnosis of the disease. Proc. Book Amer. vet. med. Ass. **91,** 167—177 (1954).

MIYAMOTO, T., K. TAKEHARA, Y. NOMURA, T. SAMEJIMA, and J. NAKAMURA: Passages of the virus of bluetongue-like disease of cattle in mice and embryonating chicken eggs. N. I. B. S. Bull. biol. Res. Tokyo **7,** 1—18 (1962—1963).

MOULTON, J. E.: Pathology of bluetongue of sheep in California. J. Amer. vet. med. Ass. **138,** 493—498 (1961).

NEITZ, W. O.: The Blesbuck *(Damaliscus albifrons)* as a carrier of heartwater and bluetongue. J. S. Afr. vet. med. Ass. **4,** 24—26 (1933).

NEITZ, W. O.: Immunological studies on bluetongue in sheep. Onderstepoort J. vet. Sci. Anim. Ind. **23,** 93—136 (1948).

NEITZ, W. O., and G. RIEMERSCHMID: The influence of solar radiation on the course of bluetongue. Onderstepoort J. vet. Sci. Anim. Ind. **20,** 29—56 (1944).

NIESCHULZ, O., G. A. H. BEDFORD, and R. M. DU TOIT: Investigations into the transmission of bluetongue in sheep during the season 1931/1932. Onderstepoort J. vet. Sci. Anim. Ind. **2,** 509—562 (1934).

OMORI, T.: Bluetongue-like disease in Japan. Bull. Off. int. Epiz. **55,** 1109—1117 (1961).

OWEN, N. C.: Investigation into the pH stability of bluetongue virus and its survival in mutton and beef. Onderstepoort J. vet. Res. **31,** 109—118 (1964).

OWEN, N. C., and E. K. MUNZ: Observations on a strain of bluetongue virus by electron microscopy. Onderstepoort J. vet. Res. **33,** 9—14 (1966).

OWEN, N. C., R. M. DU TOIT, and P. G. HOWELL: Bluetongue in cattle: Typing of viruses isolated from cattle exposed to natural infections. Onderstepoort J. vet. Res. **32,** 3—6 (1965).

PINI, A., W. COACKLEY, and H. OHDER: The adverse effect of some calf sera on the isolation and propagation of bluetongue virus in tissue culture. Arch. ges. Virusforsch. **18,** 88—95 (1966 a).

PINI, A., W. COACKLEY, and H. OHDER: Concentration of bluetongue virus in experimentally infected sheep and virus identification by immune fluorescence technique. Arch. ges. Virusforsch. **18,** 385—390 (1966 b).

PLOTKIN, S. A., B. J. COHEN, and H. KOPROWSKI: Intratypic serodifferentiation of polioviruses. Virology **15**, 473—485 (1961).

POLSON, A.: The particle size of the bluetongue virus as determined by ultra-filtration and ultra-centrifugation. Onderstepoort J. vet. Sci. Anim. Ind. **23**, 137—148 (1948).

POLSON, A., and H. M. V. VAN REGENMORTEL: A new method for determination of sedimentation constants of viruses. Virology **15**, 397—403 (1961).

PREVEC, L., and A. F. GRAHAM: Reovirus-specific polyribosomes in infected L-cells. Science **154**, 522—523 (1966).

PRICE, D. A.: The problem of bluetongue control in range sheep. Proc. U.S. Livestock Sanit. Ass. 58th Ann. Meeting, Nov., 256—259 (1954).

PRICE, D. A., and W. T. HARDY: Isolation of the bluetongue virus from Texas sheep — *Culicoides* shown to be a vector. J. Amer. vet. med. Ass. **124**, 255—258 (1954).

RICHARDS, W. P. C., and D. R. CORDY: Bluetongue virus infection: pathologic responses of nervous systems in sheep and mice. Science **156**, 530—531 (1967).

ROBERTSON, A., M. APPEL, G. L. BANNISTER, G. M. RUCKERBAUER, and P. BOULANGER: Studies on bluetongue. II. Complement-fixation activity of ovine and bovine sera. Canadian J. comp. Med. **29**, 113—117 (1965).

ROBINSON, R. M., T. L. HAILEY, C. W. LIVINGSTON, and J. W. THOMAS: Bluetongue in the desert bighorn sheep. J. Wildl. Mgmt. **31**, 165—168 (1967).

ROBINSON, R. M., C. L. STAIR, and L. P. JONES: Bluetongue in deer. Bull. Wildl. Dis. Ass. **3**, 91 (1967).

RUCKERBAUER, G. M., D. P. GRAY, A. GIRARD, G. L. BANNISTER, and P. BOULANGER: Studies on Bluetongue. V. Detection of the virus infected materials by immunofluorescence. Canad. J. comp. Med. **31**, 175—181 (1967).

SAPRE, S. N.: An outbreak of bluetongue in goats and sheep in Maharashtra State, India. Vet. Rev. **15**, 69—71 (1964).

SARWAR, M. M.: A note on bluetongue in sheep in West Pakistan. Pakist. J. Anim. Sci. **1**, 1—2 (1962).

SCHULTZ, G., and P. D. DELAY: Losses in newborn lambs associated with bluetongue vaccination of pregnant ewes. J. Amer. vet. med. Ass. **127**, 224—226 (1955).

SHATKIN, A. J., and B. RADA: Reovirus-directed RNA synthesis in infected L-cells. J. Virol. **1**, 24—35 (1967).

SHATKIN, A. J., and J. D. SIPE: Single stranded, adenine-rich RNA from purified reoviruses. Proc. nat. Acad. Sci. (Wash.) **59**, 246—253 (1968).

SHONE, D. K., D. A. HAIG, and D. G. MCKERCHER: The use of tissue culture propagated bluetongue virus for complement fixation studies on sheep sera. Onderstepoort J. vet. Res. **27**, 179—182 (1956).

SILVA, F. S.: Lingua azol au febre cattal des ovines (blue tongue). Rev. Cienc. vet. (Lisboa) **51**, 191—231 (1956).

SPREULL, J.: Report from veterinary surgeon Spreull on the result of his experiments with the malarial catarrhal fever of sheep. Agric. J. C. G. H. **20**, 469 (1902).

SPREULL, J.: Malarial catarrhal fever (Bluetongue) of sheep in South Africa. J. comp. Path. **18**, 321—337 (1905).

STUDDERT, M. J.: Sensitivity of bluetongue virus to ether and sodium deoxycholate. Proc. Soc. exp. Biol. (N.Y.) **118**, 1006—1009 (1965).

STUDDERT, M. J., J. PANGBORN, and R. B. ADDISON: Bluetongue virus structure. Virology **29**, 509—511 (1966).

SVEHAG, S.-E.: Quantitative studies of blue tongue virus in mice. Arch. ges. Virusforsch. **12**, 363—386 (1962).

SVEHAG, S.-E.: Effect of different "Contact conditions" on the bluetongue virus-antibody reaction and on the validity of the "Percentage Law". Arch. ges. Virusforsch. **12**, 678—693 (1963a).

SVEHAG, S.-E.: Thermal inactivation of bluetongue virus. Arch. ges. Virusforsch. **13**, 499—510 (1963b).

SVEHAG, S.-E.: Quantal and graded dose-responses of bluetongue virus: a comparison of their sensitivity as assay methods for neutralising antibody. J. Hyg. (Lond.) **64**, 231—244 (1966).

SVEHAG, S.-E., and J. R. GORHAM: Passive transfer of immunity to bluetongue virus from vaccinated maternal mice to their offspring. Res. vet. Sci. **4,** 109—113 (1963).

SVEHAG, S.-E., L. LEENDERTSEN, and J. R. GORHAM: Sensitivity of bluetongue virus to lipid solvents, trypsin and pH changes and its serological relationship to arboviruses. J. Hyg. (Lond.) **64,** 339—346 (1966).

TAMER, R.: Bluetongue of sheep in Hatay (Turkey) and losses over five years. Türk. vet. Hekim. dern. Derg. **19,** 542—548 (1949).

THEILER, A.: Bluetongue in sheep. Ann. Rep. Dir. Agric. Transvaal for 1904—1905, 110—121 (1906).

THEILER, A.: The inoculation of sheep against bluetongue and the results in practice. Vet. J. **64,** 600—607 (1908).

THOMAS, A. D., and W. O. NEITZ: Further observations on the pathology of bluetongue in sheep. Onderstepoort J. vet. Sci. Anim. Ind. **22,** 27—40 (1947).

VAN DEN ENDE, M., ANNE LINDER, and V. R. KASCHULA: Experiments with the Cyprus strain of bluetongue virus: Multiplication in the central nervous system of mice and complement fixation. J. Hyg. (Lond.) **52,** 155—164 (1954).

VAN ROOYEN, P. J., and K. E. WEISS: The stab-method for inoculation of fertile eggs. Bull. epiz. Dis. Afr. **7,** 75—78 (1959).

VERWOERD, D. W.: Purification and characterization of bluetongue Virus. Virology **38,** 203—212 (1969).

VERWOERD, D. W.: Proc. 1st int. Congr. Virology, Helsinki, 1968, pp. 204—207. Int. Virology I (J. L. MELNICK, ed.) Karger, Basel, München, New York, 1970.

VOSDINGH, R. A., D. O. TRAINER, and B. C. EASTERDAY: Experimental bluetongue disease in white-tailed deer. Canad. J. comp. Med. **32,** 382—387 (1968).

WELLS, E. A.: A disease resembling bluetongue occurring in topi *(Damaliscus korrigum ugandae)* in the Queen Elizabeth National Park, Uganda. Vet. Rec. **74,** 1372—1373 (1962).

YOUNG, S., and D. R. CORDY: An ovine foetal encephalopathy caused by bluetongue vaccine virus. J. Neuropath. exp. Neurol. **23,** 635—659 (1964).

ZAKI, A. H. H.: Suspected bluetongue cases in UAR. Bull. Off. int. Epiz. **64,** 667—670 (1965).

Addendum

Recent studies have shown the isolated double-stranded RNA genome to consist of ten fragments, similar but not identical in size distribution to those of reovirus [VERWOERD, D. W.: Diplornaviruses: a newly recognized group of double-stranded RNA viruses. Progr. med. Virol. **12,** 192—210 (1970); VERWOERD, D. W., H. LOUW and R. A. OELLERMANN: Characterization of bluetongue virus ribonucleic acid. J. Virol. **5,** 1—7 (1970)]. Furthermore it has been demonstrated that infection of mouse fibroblasts with blue-tongue virus leads to early inhibition of cellular protein and DNA synthesis.